What is
Medical History

What is
Medical History?

JOHN BURNHAM

polity

Copyright © John Burnham 2005

The right of John Burnham to be identified as Author of this Work has
been asserted in accordance with the UK Copyright, Designs and Patents
Act 1988.

First published in 2005 by Polity Press

Polity Press
65 Bridge Street
Cambridge CB2 1UR, UK

Polity Press
350 Main Street
Malden, MA 02148, USA

ISBN: 0-7456-3224-6
ISBN: 0-7456-3225-4 (paperback)

A catalogue record for this book is available from the British Library.

Typeset in 10.5 on 12 pt Sabon
by SNP Best-set Typesetter Ltd., Hong Kong
Printed and bound in Great Britain by TJ International Ltd, Padstow,
Cornwall

For further information on Polity, visit our website: www.polity.co.uk

Contents

Preface

This book is designed for a reader who has encountered the history of medicine for the first time and wants an introduction. The title *What is Medical History?* is therefore appropriate. Medical history is what medical historians write about. In what follows, I shall try to explain what medical historians have done and are doing. Describing their work implicitly brings up what they have not done, or have done only incompletely or imperfectly, for they have, in fact, left many opportunities for the future.

I try to suggest why study of the history of medicine is important. And I try to explain why so many people enjoy medical history and why the field is expanding so rapidly. Learning about the past of health and health care, it turns out, is a lot of fun, on many different levels. But this book, it should be clear, is primarily not about the answers that medical historians have found, but about questions.

Because this is a very brief book, I have not been able to include the usual full scholarly apparatus of notes and references. The nature of the book precludes mentioning in the text or anywhere else most of the scholars whose publications I have drawn upon. Colleagues in medical history should be able to recognize places where I allude to their findings without their needing to be named explicitly. It is, I think, a proud company to be in, and I salute and thank those many excellent scholars who, with few exceptions, I cannot mention by name.

Particularly at the end, a short introduction to the literature and sources in the field, should the reader wish to share in my excitement and that of my colleagues, may help guide the beginner into further reading or research. These clues, in fact, eventually lead to all of the authors whose work the text reflects, and many, many more. I hope that each reader will join us and share in our pleasure in finding out how people in the past went about dealing with human illnesses.

I am deeply grateful to scholars who read an early draft and made valuable suggestions for improvement: my colleagues in the Medical Heritage Center at The Ohio State University, George Paulson and Charles Wooley; Ynez V. O'Neill in the History of Medicine at UCLA; and Roberto Padilla of the Department of History at The Ohio State University.

Implicitly this book acknowledges my graduate and postdoctoral fellowship teachers, George Harmon Knoles, Merle Curti, Charles Donald O'Malley, Owsei Temkin, Ilza Veith, David Rapaport, and Roy Schafer – and three special colleague-teachers, Eric T. Carlson, Stanley Jackson, and Jacques Quen. One by one they revealed to me attractions of medical history.

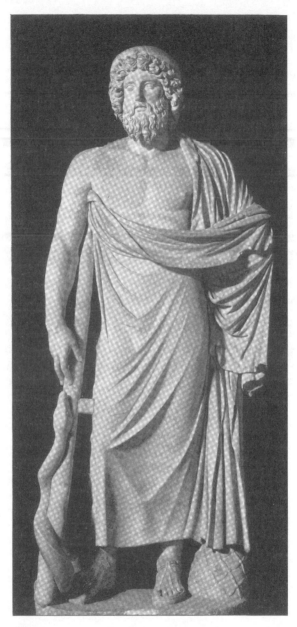

An ancient statue of the Greek god of healing, Aesculapius, with his staff, around which a snake is wrapped. Aesculapius later was taken up as a symbol of physicians in countries honoring the Western classical tradition.

Source: Eugen Holländer, *Plastik und Medizin* (1912).

Introduction

Where Medical History Came From

The work of historians of medicine and health reflects an impressive record of investigating, thinking, and writing. But the field of medical history is expanding at break-neck speed. The dynamic state of the field helps explain why both scholars and casual readers find the past of medicine and health particularly exciting.

Most specialized fields of history, such as diplomatic history, started out as aspects of general history that were refined and eventually split off. The pattern of the history of medicine was entirely otherwise. The history of medicine was at the beginning a separate and narrow field, cultivated entirely by and for physicians. Only in the twentieth century, and especially the late twentieth century, did the subject attract the interest of other kinds of historians, who then began to carry the specialized subject matter into more general social history. At the same time, they brought all aspects of social history into the history of medicine – to the point that we now generally speak of the history of medicine and health.

This recent interchange with a multiplicity of varieties of history helps explain how a subject interesting in itself has become even more attractive. The interchange also explains the end point of each of the chapters that follow below: medical history leads one to go in unexpected directions, many of which cannot now be foreseen.

How Medical History Began

The first historical accounts of the development of the lore and practice of healing had two aspects. First, the physician authors were concerned to describe and discuss the teachings of great medical writers, beginning with the classical texts of Hippocrates (ca. 460–370 BC) and Galen (AD 129–216?). The second distinctive aspect was that the purpose of the histories was to teach the views of the authors of those traditional texts written many centuries before – that is, teach them as then-current and useful medical knowledge. The history of medicine at the beginning, therefore, was but a means of presenting the eternal truths on which the practice and profession of medicine were based at that time.

This didactic goal of the first chronological accounts of medical ideas and thinkers lasted from the beginnings in the seventeenth century (the symbolic founding work was Daniel LeClerc's book, *The History of Physick*, of 1696) until the very early nineteenth century. It is true that to this day historical information from all ages about procedures and diseases still helps medical educators explain to students the content and importance of many areas of knowledge and practice. Even many lay people know, for example, the traditional technical term "placebo."

In the late eighteenth and nineteenth centuries, medical history took on new life, beyond reinforcing and explaining the classics of medicine. Medical historians of the Enlightenment period began by adopting the general idea of progress. The history of medicine therefore became a narrative in which one idea progressed to another, presumably better, idea. W. H. Williams, for example, as early as 1804 wrote *A Concise Treatise on the Progress of Medicine*. The narrative in such works was about ideas, and the ideas were associated with an author (for example, William Harvey, who published his masterpiece in 1628 and departed from the text of Galen to describe or "discover" how the blood circulates).

Then in the middle and last part of the nineteenth century, the prestige of science grew, accompanied by a hard-headed observational and experimental outlook, and the history of medicine conformed to the norms of science. Charles

Daremberg actually called his 1870 classic book *The History of Medical Science*. Thus the physicians who were writing medical history reframed their subject matter in four ways. First, they began to emphasize that progress meant not only accepting new knowledge but rejecting old ideas. Second, by focusing on medical discoveries, the historians played up the great innovators. Third, physicians' improvement of knowledge and their humanitarianism made it possible to portray medicine as a major element contributing to civilization at any point in Western history. And, fourth, by emphasizing the contributions and importance of medical activities, medical historians could use their narratives to bolster physicians' claims against non-medical practitioners and pretenders, who usually represented "errors" of the past. The medical properties of figs about which medieval physicians wrote, for example, could not be substantiated in either clinical or laboratory testing. Medical history, although still closely held by physicians, now, therefore, not only served internal teaching and professional purposes but also was used to some extent in public and political arenas (especially in Germany, where most of the writing originated).

Developing a Classic Profile

In the opening years of the twentieth century, medical historians were here and there (again, especially in Germany) making their subject a part of medical school training. Karl Sudhoff of Leipzig founded a major specialty journal for the field, and *Sudhoffs Archiv*, as it is now known, is still being published. National interest groups formed, and as early as 1920–1, an international society for the history of medicine had appeared.

As these standard institutions of a specialty field materialized, the subject matter of the history of medicine developed a classic profile that persisted as a core of the disciplinary area through most of the twentieth century (and after, for some historians). The history of medicine consisted of great doctors making discoveries and adding to knowledge. And that knowledge was understood as part of the high culture of Western civilization. Over the generations, the quality of the historical writers' research improved, but the basic narrative persisted. Even in the dark days of 1944–5, it was possible to count in a year more than 3,000 new "publications of medico-historical interest." The bulk of those writings was produced by doctors who were not gifted historians and who were almost ritually repeating, or working within, the received narrative. But among the many writers, an elite professional group made the history of medicine a high-quality, if still narrow, special field.

Especially during the 1960s, some scholars began to notice that this great-doctors-discovering narrative helped insulate the high-status medical profession from social criticism. Therefore after about 1960, even in medical history, some dissenting thinkers began to use history to attack the authority of physicians. Moreover, the medical institutions, such as hospitals, that embodied physician authority also became fair game for critical revisionist writers. Some went so far as to suggest that what passed for progress in medicine might have had undesirable side effects or contain antisocial flaws. In addition, arguments about "ethics" and "socialized medicine" on both sides of the Atlantic (and elsewhere) gave the writings of both physicians and their critics sometimes arresting overtones.

At that point, scholars in the field began to explore a factor that had been becoming more and more obvious since the end of the nineteenth century: what happened in medicine had profound effects, whether in social policy and economics or in the individual lives that were affected fundamentally by medical care. What was at the time most urgent in the eyes of many public-spirited people, including reformers within the medical profession, was people who could not get medical care.

The Coming of the Social Historians

But already by the 1920s, and especially the 1930s, another group of historians had begun to concern themselves with the history of medicine. These were the highly trained social historians. At first only a handful in the field of medical history, the numbers of scholars grew rapidly, especially in the decades after World War II. The physicians who in the early twentieth century were writing the best medical history were bright people. They perceived at once that they could learn a lot from professional historians about the standards of historical research and writing, and they did so. But their efforts only added to the new look that medical history was taking on, as PhD historians rather than doctors of medicine began to flood into the field. It is the results of the work of both groups, influenced by general intellectual changes, that constitute the subject matter of this book.

The first social historians of medicine were part of the so-called New History movement that came out of the United States between the world wars. Beginning in the 1960s and 1970s, they were joined by a number of British historians interested in the history of the common people, and by a similar group of Continental scholars who also wrote about common people and who raised questions about changes in social structures in the past. Although these historians often wrote with strong critical and social agendas, they shared a concern with broadening the kinds of sources that medical historians used and the kinds of people who would figure in their analyses. And for those who started out in general social history, the history of medicine provided a wonderfully rich area in which to explore various advanced historical problems and theories – particularly, how do we get knowledge about the actions and cultures of ordinary people of the past, and how good is that information?

The social historians were especially valuable as they called attention to the history of social institutions within which healing flourished and, most importantly, to the doctor–patient relationship. By focusing on patients in what was called from-the-bottom-up history (as opposed to a narrative of elite medical thinkers and leaders), they brought many new dimensions to the history of medicine, as Christopher Lawrence (concisely) and many other scholars (at length) have commented.[1] These historians even pointed out that sick people often chose medical practitioners other than physicians. And the social historians brought additional interest to the field. As historian Joan Lane observes, "The social history of medicine ... is, by any standards, the history of every inhabitant. As we all experience birth, illness, ageing, and death, we all become patients at one time or another, in the care of various branches of medicine, as did most of our ancestors."[2]

Even histories of technical medicine, written usually by physicians, were affected by the new questioning and new times. How did people's ideas of health and illness change? Technology had become so important in medical practice that much of the recent history could borrow from another history specialty group, the historians of technology. Or one could talk about the end product of technology as did nineteenth-century writers of sea stories and twentieth-century writers of science fiction: one could follow the story without having to understand the principles by which devices worked.

A General Framework: Medicalization vs. Demedicalization

As one takes perspective on the way in which the field of the history of medicine came to such a flourishing state by the beginning of the twenty-first century, it becomes clear that one overarching theme embraces all of the various changes and tensions in this area of study. All of the writers, whether technical and intellectual or using one of the sociocultural history approaches, are concerned with the forces of medicalization and demedicalization.

Medicalization, according to some writers, was an attempt by a medical establishment, using ideas out of the world of healing, to impose a pattern of social control on a population. In every sizable society, as the historical record shows, healers – clinicians – worked to expand their effectiveness, their clientele, and their social influence. They sought to have their expertise recognized beyond the family or immediate social group. In every society, too, many people worked to defend themselves or their social territories from the influence of the healers, from being medicalized. The dissenters operated with ideas that were not part of a medical outlook. If someone – one's self or a friend or relative – was ill, they wanted to pray for the patient. Or they wanted to use folk remedies validated by tradition, not new-fangled vaccinations. Or they wanted to define some human quirk as not a disease process but as a moral or social or animistic condition.

Medicalization was generally not a deliberate program in a culture. Sometimes it had existed for a long time, as in China from very ancient times diet was profoundly medicalized. Foods served medical and health purposes. Each season had foods that might bring illness (as with a cold) or health, as the flesh of a certain animal would make one strong in wintertime. To this day, there is a particular dish, "medicine chicken."

Historians most often notice changes in the extent to which medical thinking shaped life. The social process of medicalization was, indeed, most marked at times when much social stress was evident. And the process took many forms. In simply the perception and naming of a new disease, like scarlet fever or Legionnaire's disease, clinicians and biomedical scientists medicalized a small part of life, moving appearances and subjective feelings into a named medical category. Language itself revealed how many ways a condition could move in or out of the medical realm. At one time, good-looking people were often plump or stout. Later the same individuals became "overweight" and possibly the subject of medical concern. Personal lifestyle could become a "health risk" (medicalization) or could defiantly be the way one wished to behave (demedicalization). In the late twentieth century, moving sexuality out of the realm of medicine and into the realm of morals was a marked form of demedicalization.

In recent times, cleanliness became a product of social standards and economic interest, not health. Manufacturers and marketers of soaps thus unwittingly demedicalized a health dictum – be clean and healthy. Yet it is a sign of irony as well as complexity that the advertisers of cleaning products often employed medical rationales and metaphors to get people to buy their products – to the extent, for example, of inventing a new common-knowledge disorder, halitosis.

At least part of the time, pressures and initiatives to medicalize one human concern or another came from those, like the advertisers, outside the ranks of the healers. Indeed, whole populations embraced medical thinking eagerly, as Robert Nye and others point out.[3] Beginning in the early modern period, enthusiasts used medical approaches to demystify many phenomena. Perhaps the most famous case was the campaign of physician Johann Weyer and others in the late sixteenth century to explain witchcraft in terms of naturalistic mental illness. Many people, then and later, found explanations offered by medical thinkers, in terms of physical nature, superior to explanations based variously on tradition and superstition.

Medicalization often went far beyond group power or personal choice. Very early in the history of Europeanized societies, creative writers employed medical metaphors. Institutions could be sick. Reformers could act as physicians to society. In interpersonal relations, a person could be a pain in the neck or some other part of the anatomy. So one could take the very construction of the world in which one lived and see how much it contained what one knew, directly or indirectly, of medicine. Indeed, one could weigh how much money was being spent on health care (as opposed to other things) and could think that even the economy was too much, or not enough, medicalized. What was one to make of the Americans, who at the opening of the twenty-first century spent about 14 percent of the national income on health care?

Questions of public health – particularly the effects and controls of pollution – quickly passed from the hands of physicians and biomedical scientists into the hands of politicians and citizens' groups, transformed into new terms that, in this case, demedicalized the issues. Most urgently, different types of deviant behavior have, over time, passed from clergy to lawyers to physicians and back again. Historians have put much effort into sorting out exactly which profession was handling crime, suicide, madness, and various apparently bodily ailments at different times. As Janet Golden has pointed out, demedicalization was more than just undoing medicalization. It could represent a force in itself.[4]

My intent is to show as much as possible the richness of the ways in which the history of medicine leads one into many different areas of inquiry suggested by the processes of medicalization and demedicalization. To this end, I suggest that it is most useful to conceive of the history of medicine as the simultaneous and intertwining working of five great dramas. Each of these dramas is built on intriguing work by scholars. But each historical drama remains suggestive and open-ended. And each one can be read in terms of the ways in which both historians and their subjects were caught up in the tensions between medicalization and demedicalization.

The metaphor of a drama has another advantage. In each drama, one can focus on a general problem, such as the doctor–patient relationship, or the argument between heroic interventionist therapy and supportive, gentle treatment. Or one can focus on a narrative and development through time. A drama can thus contextualize either a topical or a chrono-logical historical discussion.

The primary structure in the dramas remains the idea of the progress of Western medicine and medical institutions – and how this "progress" translated into medicalization. It would be an error to lose sight of the continuing centrality of this narrative and the subplots associated with it. But many historians now focus on what the narrative looked like to others, particularly those outside of the Europeanized world as, for example, traditional Japanese healers had to adapt first to Chinese medicine and then to Dutch medicine. Such schol-ars offer a variety of different versions of the drama.

Historians therefore have a growing awareness of parallel and often interacting dramas in medical systems in non-Western cultures. When that awareness is added to the expan-sion, intensification, and localization of investigations of the central narrative, the history of medicine takes on still addi-tional dimensions of open-endedness.

Yet the history of medicine is like other history in that scholars continue to search for evidence – evidence that will perfect the narrative in each drama, and evidence that will resolve controversies that give a special edge to following the story of what happened.

The First Drama

The Healer

In every known society, someone plays the role of healer.

Any organism injured, or attacked by a hostile life form such as a bacterium, will mobilize defenses to try to maintain life. Animals will lick wounds, rest, seek water, and undertake other healing actions. But human beings typically have brought in an outside party, a healer, to attend and treat a patient. Or humans could even create a whole social structure to define and correct illness – now clumsily known as a health care delivery system.

Healers and Priests

For some time, Western thinkers imagined that modern societies evolved from societies that were like the "primitive" societies that explorers had discovered. Typically in such societies, the healer was the "witch doctor," a familiar, stereotypical figure who used religious ceremonies and weird substances to cure someone who was ill.

Scholars no longer believe that modern medicine had its origins in the practice of the witch doctor or medicine man. Nevertheless, information about healers in very different cultures, from the shaman dealing with broken taboos or witchcraft to the most advanced specialist in our own tribal setting,

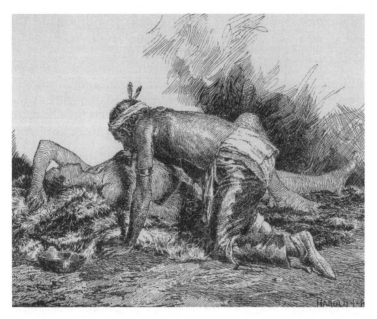

Detail of a contemporary drawing of a nineteenth-century Ojibwa (American Plains Indian) shaman sucking disease out of a patient's body, apparently through a hollow reed.

Source: Seventh Annual Report of the Bureau of Ethnology to the Secretary of the Smithsonian Institution, 1885–6.

can expose and highlight the very basic constituents of the act of healing. In particular, shaman figures show that a healer plays – and played – a priestly role.

To this day in most societies, when a physician enters an examining room, he or she still carries some aura of priestliness sensed by patient, by paramedicals, and implicitly by the physician himself or herself. The very idea that the physician plays a role has encouraged literary artists to explore doctoring as performance on the stage of society.

What is particularly striking about the overlap with priestliness is the persistence of the universal, essential ceremony in all kinds of healing. First the healer has to make a diagnosis as to what, if anything, ails the patient. The second part of the ceremony (and the most uncertain) is the prognosis: what will be the future course of the disease process? In ancient times, when people had little expectation of cure, the reputation of a physician often depended upon his (*sic*) ability to predict the course of the patient's illness. The next part of the ceremony was, of course, the prescription. Generations of practitioners have found that they must provide some prescription, if only a sugar pill. Any physician who does not give the patient a prescription will lose patients, for, typically, a patient will feel deprived if he or she has to depart without a prescription. Finally comes the bill. The universality of this concluding part of the ceremony is testified to by the anonymous author of a children's song that rhymes "bill" with "pill." The connection – indeed, the whole ceremony – has seemed natural to many generations in many different national cultures.

Medical historians continue to trace the elements in the medical ceremony as those elements changed over time. How did physicians decide to categorize and understand the symptoms and make a diagnosis? Some years ago, for example, the French philosopher Michel Foucault suggested that the physician's "gaze" could make a great deal of difference in the way he or she conceptualized what was happening to the patient. Indeed, Foucault suggested that the "gaze" might even involve sociopolitical relationships. Or in prognosis, simply the struggle of past medical figures to understand a disease process continues to attract writers of one narrative after another. Why are the fever patterns in malaria so regular? The history of therapeutics likewise evokes the most lively interest. And physicians' fees engender a fascination that is hard to explain – but many writers still try. One, for example, years ago suggested that the record for a physician's fee was that earned in 1768 by the British physician, Thomas Dimsdale, for inoculating Catherine the Great and her son for smallpox: £10,000 cash, an annual pension of £5,000, and a Russian baronetcy and the title of councilor of state (to get the equivalent figures for today, one should multiply by perhaps 100).

Even in the person of the witch doctor, however, it is possible to discern one of the basic questions in the history of medicine. Where did the healing power of the doctor come from? For some witch doctors, the power lay in themselves, in their special relationship to the gods. Raymond Prince quotes a Yoruban shaman in Nigeria who, after his father's death, took up healing by divination. "I had a dream. I saw my father, and he took me to the box of instruments . . . When I awakened in the morning, I felt happy and decided to try it . . . When I have a difficult case, my father comes to me in my dream to help me."[1] As late as the nineteenth century, the physician's personal authority, historians point out, was the most important factor in the practice of most medicine.

But other witch doctors developed their power not because of personality and charisma as much as through their knowledge and skill in manipulating and using nature, in knowing how to bring the body into harmony with the environment, in knowing which natural materials, such as herbs, had healing power. And many shamans were skilled in foretelling the course of a disease. Thus even in the religious or superstitious aspect of medicine, another basic of medicine appeared: the healer had special knowledge, and he or she could pass this body of knowledge down to other healers. The knowledge could be either spiritual or natural – or both.

People in the ancient civilizations that gave rise to Western practices appeared to be comfortable with the interchangeability and confusion between natural and religious means of healing. Physicians, who were clearly identified in those societies, functioned on the basis of both religious and empirical beliefs. In the Code of Hammurabi (ca. 1750 BC), the physician was identified as such. From perhaps 3000 BC in Babylonia, we have the personal seal of a physician, a light gray alabaster cylinder inscribed:

> O Edinmugi, Servant of the god Girra, who helps mothers in childbed, Ur-Lugaledina the physician is thy servant.

From ancient Egypt there has survived a portrait of a physician who is actually identified by name, but the term "physician" there, too, included religious as well as strictly medical functioning. A few medical papyri have survived, and they show how – even aside from the process of mummification – medicine involved religious ceremonies along with empirical procedures. In the 1550 BC Ebers Papyrus, a prescription for treating a burn demonstrates how intertwined were the religious and natural approaches to healing, with an incantation specified as part of the prescription:

> "O thou son of god, Horus! There be Fire in the Land! Though there be water there or not now, the Water is in thy Mouth, the Nile is at thy Feet when thou comest to quench the Fire."
> To be spoken over
> Milk-of-a-Woman-who-has-Borne-a-Son.
> Cake
> Ram's Hair
> Apply to the Burn.

Historians disagree concerning the extent to which religious and medical practitioners were distinct in Egypt, and scholars are still examining the structure of ideas in surviving documents. But in classical Greek civilization, the identities of the priest and the physician became clearly separated, although both remained in the healing business. Medical historians have reconstructed the activities of the priests in the temples of Aesculapius, the demi-god of healing. The patient would come to the temple and make appropriate sacrifices and pay the priests. Then the patient would sleep in the abaton, an open arcade facing the temple courtyard. During the night, the god in a dream would come to the patient, often in the form of a snake, and tell the patient how to be healed.

Grateful patients who were cured often left testimonies carved in stone:

> Hagestratus with headaches. He suffered from insomnia on account of headaches. When he came to the Abaton he fell asleep and saw a dream. It seemed to him that the god cured him of his headaches and, making him stand up naked, taught him the lunge used in the pancratium. When day came he departed well, and not long afterwards he won in the pancratium at the Nemean games.

Aesculapius was the son of Apollo, and he had two daughters, Hygeia and Panacea. From the symbolism of classical Greece came the symbol of the physician, the caduceus, which features a snake, representing Aesculapius. Physicians who valued the traditions of their guild have lovingly traced these remnants of priestly healing as a legitimate part of their professional ancestry.

Naturalism in Ancient Medicine

Those interested in ancient medicine have, like other scholars concerned with that period, worked with finding written records, with translating the texts, with fitting fragments together, and with inferring social and other contexts of healing. Any of these achievements can give rise to lively controversy. Is the fragment authentic? When was the text composed?

The most intense interest of medical historians has focused on the naturalistic version of ancient Greek healing, which constituted the medical teaching and practice of that day. What happened was that in the eighth and seventh centuries BC, Greek philosophers began to distinguish a world – nature – that functioned when the gods were not actively interfering. Slowly, healers who had been using Mediterranean folk medicine and empirical treatments began to conceptualize illness and the body as part of nature. They consequently believed that they could understand nature and to some extent manipulate nature to the end of curing diseases. They were not so much secularizing religious healing (as some scholars have held) as setting up a secular alternative.

The symbol of this new type of medicine, to which traditional scholars traced later Western medicine, was a teacher from the eastern Mediterranean island of Cos, Hippocrates. We know of him because of some writings, customarily referred to as the writings of Hippocrates. Scholars have determined that "the Hippocratic corpus" of writings was a collection of not necessarily consistent texts by numerous different authors, mostly from the fifth and fourth centuries BC. As with all classical texts, experts of course still disagree about what elements went into the corpus, and when – as well as how each passage should be interpreted and understood. The total body of writing, however, has served to inspire physicians ever since because of the common sense, shrewd clinical observation, and broad outlook of "Hippocrates."

What most notably marked the whole corpus was a surprisingly thoroughgoing naturalism. Historians like to quote the passage on epilepsy, "the falling sickness," which was known as the sacred disease because of the direct hand the gods presumably had in causing someone to be afflicted: "It is thus with regard to the disease called Sacred: it appears to me to be nowise more divine nor more sacred than other diseases but has a natural cause from which it originates like other affections" – and Hippocrates mentions as examples fevers, madness, and other problems that, as far as medicine was concerned, were natural in origin.

Hippocrates was of course not the only medical teacher. In both Greek and Roman times, a large number of schools, or sects, practiced and taught different styles of medicine. Some emphasized the pneuma, or spirit, that nevertheless could be treated physically. Others emphasized traditional remedies. And some were eclectics who took doctrines from all sects. Moreover, the sects, including the Hippocratic, often had strong interrelations with other classical thinkers. The second giant of ancient medicine, Galen, practicing notably in Rome in the first century, for example drew heavily on the philosopher Aristotle. Historians have endless problems trying, on limited evidence, to reconstruct the genealogy as well as the history and meaning of medical thinking in classical times. And as they get involved in the ancient texts, scholars not infrequently find themselves starting to take the part of particular participants in the debates between one sect of healers and another!

Practice and Profession

Beyond the great division between priestly and naturalistic healing in ancient times, there was another shift. According to Owsei Temkin, Greek physicians at the beginning worked from existing traditions, so that treatment consisted of applying predetermined formulas to individual patients, with an emphasis on set procedure. By about the fifth century BC, perhaps the time of Hippocrates, practice came more and more to consist of the individual efforts of the healer, applied to an individual patient. This emphasis on doctor–patient relationships and even on ethics has attracted any number of classical scholars.[2] The new type of practice, as Heinrich von Staden, another historian, points out, could even involve esthetics and public relations, as attention shifted from the religious and moral fault of the patient for being sick (common in many religions and in "primitive" healing) to the responsibility of the physician. In the Hippocratic text *On Fractures*, the author observes that even if it would be better technically to put a splint on top of a broken leg, to the non-physician, "it is more persuasive that the [physician] is less in error, if a splint is placed underneath."[3]

The Oath of Hippocrates illustrates how texts and traditions from ancient times continue to agitate historians. This traditional oath for initiates was one of many used by different schools of physicians, and the attribution to Hippocrates is spurious. The oath specifies that the doctor pledges to honor his (*sic*) teacher and keep his secrets. The doctor also will follow ethical standards such as keeping the patients' confidences, not taking advantage of patients sexually, and not furnishing poisons for evil purposes. The initiate also swore not to help in attempted abortions.

Scholars eventually showed that, despite tradition, this oath only appeared long after Hippocrates, and it flourished because it suited people with various ideas about ethics. Then, more recently, this earlier scholarship came under attack, and some scholars held the oath to be earlier and more universally respected than had been believed. And at the same time as this recent scholarship appeared, medical students started to refuse to take the traditional oath because it contained elements unsuited for modern times. The suitability of requiring medical graduates to recite the oath was still being seriously debated in the twenty-first century.

The issues around the Oath of Hippocrates and the history of medical ethics were all part of the great drama in which physicians over the centuries struggled to win professional recognition and status. In this drama, the protagonists were not so much individuals like Galen or, say, William Osler, the author of a defining medical textbook first published in 1892, as they were a group collectively struggling for authority, status, and income. Indeed, one gauge of the extent to which societies were medicalized is the extent to which physicians there developed social recognition for their profession.

In the middle of the twentieth century, when physicians were at the height of their public recognition, medicine was the model profession. At that point, many scholars tried to figure out what it meant to be a professional, and the definition from that period has colored understanding of the past of physicians as professionals. Historians of early modern period medicine have particularly objected to applying the sociological formulations of the 1950s to the complicated and changing layers of trained and untrained healers active in the sixteenth and seventeenth centuries. Moreover, in the nineteenth and twentieth centuries, academic medicine taught in the universities was often of a different texture from the medicine that practitioners worked with every day. Yet some of the sociologists' formulations continue to be helpful in understanding what happened at different times in the past.

In all societies, professionals were typically those who dealt with the gray, uncertain areas of human existence: a person's personal relationship to nature (physicians), to other people (lawyers), and to God (priests). The stereotypical witch doctor was an all-round professional who could handle interpersonal and religious problems as well as illnesses. But, as historian Vern Bullough pointed out, it was with the coming of the medieval university, with faculties of law and theology as well as medicine, that professions and professionals developed in a way that moderns might recognize. At that time, university-trained physicians gained the right to practice as members of an exclusive guild because local authorities recognized them and their special social role, just as other exclusive guilds functioned in medieval society.[4]

Between medieval times and the twentieth century, members of the guilds of physicians in the West struggled to gain an ever more advantageous position in society. That they often did not succeed is part of the story. But the later characterization of an ideal profession helps raise questions so that it is easier to understand how, beginning in the medieval period, physicians worked together for social leverage. A profession in the mid-twentieth century (1) functioned on the basis of a systematic body of knowledge; (2) sold expert opinion, and the customer was not always right; (3) enjoyed various community sanctions, often with licensing and exclusive licensing; (4) observed ethical codes enforced by colleagues so as to keep the group innocuous to society; (5) functioned within a subculture, typically marked by professional associations; (6) took a morally neutral stance toward clients, one that was non-profit and humanitarian, with fee collection kept separate from the service. Finally, (7) implicitly a professional held relatively high social status.[5]

In classical times, physicians did not meet such a test for a profession. Physicians were not only divided on issues of knowledge and approaches, but they had a social status roughly equal only to that of other artisans, like carpenters. Moreover, they were crassly commercial, often wandering about hawking, not their wares, but their cures and services. Even the Hippocratic corpus contains continuous attacks on the practices of other physicians. Galen pictured most of the physicians of his time as ignorant and avaricious, and he compared them to the robbers who lived in the hills and preyed on travelers. But a number of historians have pointed out that at least in Rome, authorities awarded government appointments that gave recognition to some physicians, and well-informed people could recognize trained and accomplished healers. Altogether, what happened in the actual practice of medicine and the condition of ancient physicians remains a contentious and very interesting area of research.

Stimulated by the anachronous twentieth-century model, historians of the post-Roman West have examined medical practice for signs of self-policed ethics, a systematic body of knowledge, and licensing. These historians have insisted that, in their own way, physicians in Renaissance guilds and early modern societies did have a profession, but the profile differed from that of the twentieth century and was tied to the conditions of the times, whatever they were. As late as the eighteenth century, for example, the aristocratic officers of the Austrian army could have physicians under their command whipped if their practice was unsatisfactory. Even in that context, the identity of the physician as a special figure in society, one who could commit malpractice, was clearly recognized. So tensions continue in historical writing between a later, universal idea of profession, on the one hand, and the extent to which time and place determined the ways in which healers were identified and functioned in their social contexts, on the other.

Struggles for Recognition

The tensions define the continuing drama in which physicians as a distinguishable group claimed to have a special social role and yet fell short, to various degrees, in gaining specific social recognition. Or sometimes won it.

The drama had many versions. The most obvious came in formal, legal measures: the chartering of various Royal Societies in Britain, the stipulation of fee levels by numerous local authorities, the inclusion of physician compensation in German social insurance, the repeal (!) of licensing laws in all of the states of the United States (as well as quite independently in Colombia) in the middle of the nineteenth century, followed, decades later, by a struggle to reinstitute licensing. Of great contemporary interest is the way in which, in these struggles, professional institutions formally or informally operated at various times to exclude various types of practitioners: foreigners, minority groups, lower-class people, and – above all – women. Or sectarians, faith healers, and similar untrained or unorthodox practitioners.

Some historians have made drama of the evident ultimate success of the medical profession. Overall standards of practice rose. As basically caring and philanthropic people, physicians as professionals came to represent the prosocial and humanitarian forces of a modernizing society. Other historians have used the drama of more and better professionalization as the continuing triumph and functioning of cruel social climbing, in which narrative interest comes from the struggles of those whom the professionals marginalized and excluded and those whom physicians ignored, whether people of color, or native and folk healers, or workers and farmers without social insurance.

Historians recently have examined the role of high status – particularly how scientific physicians and their medical institutions functioned in the processes of imperialism. It is striking that in South and East Asia, where guilds of healers already existed, when Western medicine came in, according to some historians the status of the indigenous professional healers went up.

Beginning in the late nineteenth century, the process of professionalization operated not only in modernizing societies but in a context of increasing bureaucratization. Therefore the profession of medicine – now the model profession – took on the appearance of progressing, and in more than a superficial sense. In this world of increasing organization, it is no wonder that the narrative of the progress of the medical profession became and remains privileged. It is no wonder, either, that historians projected backward onto earlier times a course of steady improvement. And one can still trace the drama of the rise of the profession even as one tries to tease out the increasingly bureaucratic elements in health care.

The history of the modern Western profession derives much of its dramatic quality precisely from orthodox physicians' righteous and self-righteous struggles against quacks, sectarians, and commercial nostrum dealers. And most intriguing were the efforts of doctors as professionals to claim territory not only from clearly alternative and marginal physician groups but also from other professionals and semi-professionals, particularly lawyers and the clergy, as well as midwives, nurses, and psychologists. These other professionals and would-be professionals in their turn were attempting to claim territory from the medical profession. Some writers of the last part of the twentieth century even were projecting substantial victories of these often-economic forces of demedicalization, as in F. J. Ingelfinger's famous 1976 editorial, "Deprofessionalizing the Profession," in the *New England Journal of Medicine*: "A profession ... suffers when suspicion and distrust replaces its fiduciary image, and when commercialism supersedes other, less selfish motives."

Organized physicians were thus pitted against two forces. The first consisted of people who resisted any new medical influence or medical thinking or any other aspect of medicalization. The second force constituted those who actively wanted to demedicalize one or more aspects of society.

Many scholars have taken a skeptical perspective on the drama of clashing professional claims or turf wars. Indeed, the identities and agendas of healers were for many centuries so diverse that medicalization may be an inappropriate concept for eras before modernization became a major force. Several church edicts in medieval times forbade priests to practice medicine, but many dispensations were granted. Into the eighteenth century, many clergy of all sects practiced medicine. So did others who could read the same medical works the doctors did, medical texts that can still be identified.

Many historians therefore give special attention to the history of healing and healers without regard to formal or even social qualifications. Indeed, in Europeanized societies and in others, recognized physicians and other healers often used the same therapies, such as bleeding, and many times the rationales or theories were also the same. It was not unusual in medieval times to find a blacksmith who had a sideline in bone setting. For the early modern period, scholars have often succeeded in privileging the activities of non-physician healers right alongside those of formally trained physicians. Many historians can define a healthy medical pluralism not only in Europe but, for example, in Latin American cultures in which many varieties of *curanderos*, trained and untrained folk healers, usually empirics (working on the basis of unsystematic experience), are represented by a very large historical literature.

Marginalization and Exclusion

Not all scholars, however, accept an undiscriminating equating of healers. Even more do not agree that in later periods all healers were fulfilling the same functions, and these historians continue to write about a hierarchy in which different types of healers occupied different niches. Indeed, such historians could argue that the actions and teachings of elites in medicine had disproportionate effects on the societies and times in which they functioned.

But once one starts in on the alternatives to formally trained physicians, the opportunities for historians grow, as was particularly obvious in the 1980s and 1990s. Over the centuries, folk healing alone took as many forms as there were folk, with roots in family and community traditions, occultisms, and superstitions. When combined with rational and official teachings, broadly unconventional medicine appeared in almost endless guises, and, in addition, as historian Robert Jütte observes, "marked national, regional and cultural differences . . . compound the extraordinary diversity of alternative practices."[6] Indeed, beyond the material substances that different practitioners used, how many ways were there to "touch" someone in a healing way?

Scholars have been able to build on a traditional literature about people of various times who were in fact those whom regular physicians attacked as dangerous to people's health or as business rivals. Those slowly excluded from practice have fascinated even people who are complicit in the exclusion. Hydropaths, for example, who advocated water, taken both internally and externally, look appealing to modern eyes when the alternatives were much harsher practices and when many practitioners dispensed particularly harmful substances, like the purgative mercurial chloride (calomel).

The traditional term of denunciation for an alternative healer was "quack." A quack was someone who defrauded a patient by pretending to have medical knowledge but in fact made money by dispensing some substance or procedure the quack knew, or at least suspected, was not effective, such as "snake oil," bread pills, or bone manipulation. Quacks were often colorful characters who, by imitating the forms (as opposed to the science) of medical practice, suggested what popular understanding of those forms was.

Many healers, however, believed in their nostrums. Sincere nostrum vendors are hard to distinguish from empirics, who encountered what they believed to be a natural cure and earnestly peddled it in the hope of improving the lot of humankind. Such a sincere healer was Elisha Perkins, who in the 1790s gained transatlantic fame by discovering the power of two metal "tractors," which were pointed metal objects held in the hand of the healer. He had such faith in his therapy that he lost his life trying to save victims of the yellow fever epidemic in New York in 1799, when he contracted the disease himself.

This type of sincere healer therefore ranged from the regularly trained physician who believed that he or she had found a successful treatment, to credulous lay people who discovered their own supposed powers, to those who invoked supernatural means. Mixed in at all times with quacks and empirics were traditional faith healers, whose charisma could act on some patients with such force as to effect a detectable, and impressive, improvement, like the cures produced by Valentine Greatrakes, the seventeenth-century Irish "stroker" who treated the ill by touching them. The entire range of practitioner has flourished in Western societies since the beginning of history.

Some historians have been drawn in by the activities of the varieties of healers and have examined the processes by which boundaries did or did not exist, and why. Clerics who simultaneously dispensed medical advice and religious attention were a relatively simple case. Medical sects of the nineteenth century (quite different from those of the ancient world) present a different problem. Historians have written with both sympathy and skepticism about homeopaths (originated by a regular medical physician in Germany), botanics and eclectics (growing out of the teachings of several American non-physician empirics), hydropaths (having an origin with a non-physician German), and, later, osteopaths (originated by an American empiric). Followers of these sects numbered in the millions. When advocates of the medicine of one sect or another denounced regular medical practitioners (often very effectively), they seemed to be opposing medicalization. But since members of the sects used the forms of medicine –

the medical ceremony, the title of "doctor," professional associations – they could also serve as facilitators of medicalization. In either case, scholars have avidly written about the internal and sociocultural histories of all of the sects. Scholars have also paid particular attention to the explicit campaigns of regular physicians to marginalize and delegitimate rival medical systems. In the United States in the nineteenth century, physicians could be sanctioned for even associating with irregular physicians. The extreme case was a physician in the state of New York in the nineteenth century who was removed from the medical society for associating with a homeopathic physician. It happened that the homeopath in question was his wife.

Campaigns of exclusion and marginalization, whether of the early modern period or the nineteenth century and after, of course acquire their special significance because they have served as vivid and understandable models of the means by which dominant groups carried out the exercise of power and the struggle for social leverage. The story can become more complicated. As some historians have pointed out, it is not clear that at all times and in all places physicians were in a position to exercise power or even inadvertently oppress people.

The processes were even more complex when there were already healers on the margins. Moreover, practitioners existed within the medical profession itself who in one way or another constituted a stratum of society decidedly lower than that of the better-trained physicians – in Germany, *sekundär Ärzte* (secondary physicians); a similar group in France, the *officiers de santé*; or in Russia the *feldshers* who practiced among the peasants. Indeed, in the fourteenth century, the Korean state trained a special group of women with low social status to provide health care for women. The East India Company for a time in the nineteenth century trained a group specifically called "native doctors" to work in the absence of European physicians.

In addition, and most notably, not only nurse practitioners but midwives were part of the health care delivery system in many places for long periods of time. And so were all of the paramedical personnel who became part of the systems, including nurses and medical technicians. Were they not healers? Historians thrive examining such borderland areas.

There were too, over the ages, many wise people in every family and community whom citizens consulted. Mark Twain (Samuel Clemens) recalled from his boyhood in the mid-nineteenth century that "Every woman was a doctor; and gathered her own medicines in the woods, and knew how to compound doses that would stir the vitals of a cast-iron dog." Some neighborhood healers had formal education, but most were simply those who observed keenly and possessed common sense. In the neo-romantic late twentieth century, these wise people and folk healers became attractive subjects for historians. The wise people were particularly interesting because they often were women who were among those excluded from the ranks of formal practitioners. Some were of course midwives, and midwives were usually neither poor nor ignorant. Others, both women and men, simply embodied "the voice of experience." And they provided, particularly, alternatives to regular medicine, even when they were sympathetic to physicians' viewpoints and reinforced the forms of medicalization.

One of the recent great improvements in medical history has consisted of investigating the ways in which the power of ideas about gender shaped healing practices. These investigations typically started out as exposés of the ways in which women were excluded from the medical profession or oppressed in other ways (for example in their roles as nurses) by male physicians. The drama of the first woman medical school graduate, Elizabeth Blackwell (MD 1849), remains fresh – and revealing – in all of the obstacles and harassment that she had to overcome. Similar stories from Continental Europe also have surfaced. Such narratives were soon followed by a number of pioneer works celebrating the theretofore largely ignored accomplishments of female physicians, midwives, and nurses, emphasizing their contributions and claiming for them a just place in medical history.

Healing and Philanthropy

Later historians broadened these inquiries and made them more general. Writers found that male-dominant societies of the past still had special roles for women, and one that was particularly general was to give care, especially care for the sick. The relationship between women who played this special role, even when formalized into nursing practice in the nineteenth century, and that of the male physician, it is now clear, was not all one-sided. But historians have gone further. They point out that, as with the wise old women of a community, caring and healing were closely related, and male healers, even prestigious physicians, could play an essentially feminine role. The aspirations of physicians in the nineteenth century to attend childbirth, for example, openly attracted scorn for "male midwives," implicitly recognizing the traditions of gender.

Part of the shaping tradition of the profession came to be the idea that a physician should give care without regard to fees. Practitioners' obituaries frequently mentioned the fact that the deceased had given care to those in need, including care without compensation. "He" was caregiver to the community – clearly a feminine function. It is easy to see why some historians argue that the philanthropic element in medical care was essentially based on traditional female roles.

According to the Spanish historian Pedro Laín Entralgo, one can trace the idealization of the relation of the physician to the patient back to ancient Greek ideas of friendship – each party should view the other as a friend.[7] The physician, however, had a double loyalty. He (*sic*) was supposed to love not just humanity and the patient but medicine as an art or technique. In medieval times, religion reshaped the responsibilities of the physician. He (*sic* again) began to have an obligation to go beyond mere healing and to console and comfort the patient. The physician was to deal not just with those who might be cured, but with those who were incurable or were dying. This was a significant extension of a physician's duties, and it clearly represented a philanthropic dimension of medicalization, because the obligation of the physician to treat and comfort poor people without cost was spelled out. So consolation and charity, along with love of technique, became part of the healing ideal in Western medicine.

Many historians have recorded instances in which healers fell far short of the ideal. Such accounts can reinforce the ideal. The times when healers of all kinds showed greed are innumerable. Fear, too, often played a decisive part in determining the behavior of physicians and others – whether fear of informal community condemnation that could become dangerous in the early modern era, or fear of malpractice lawyers in the West in the last part of the twentieth century. Indeed, so many historians have taken the role of negative moralizers that it may be that medical history is neglecting the many practitioners of all kinds who treated patients when no fee or payment could be expected, who taught or lectured on health without compensation, who made great sacrifices for research or treatment in a variety of settings, including religious establishments, slums, areas devastated by epidemics and catastrophes, and hostile climates and cultures. All aspects of healers' activities in the past supply material for the historian.

Biography

How to understand healers of the past? One basic approach, and one that became popular again at the end of the twentieth century, is biography. Biography is a special category in and of itself, different from history. Yet biography can contain much good history, and historians use the specifics of biography both to explore and to explain what happened in the past.

Physicians and other healers contribute and contributed mostly intangible products. Therefore biography can serve to record the achievements of a lifetime. Many physicians have left autobiographical accounts as a way of claiming a place in history, and many biographers have used narratives of a life for the same purpose. Obviously both biography and autobiography can work to make historical claims (the most famous cases perhaps are: who was responsible for introducing surgical anesthesia in the 1840s, and who devised insulin for diabetic patients in the 1920s – both of which questions continue to be controversial). And, one should note in fairness, not all biography is necessarily sympathetic to the subject!

Or historians can use biography to try to convey what the practice of medicine or other healing was like in a particular age. In such a case, the biographee need not be especially prominent but rather should represent, as either an average or an ideal, what the work of caring for patients was like, whether in ancient India, sixteenth-century Britain, or mid-twentieth-century west Africa. For a great many scholars, the heart of medical history remains uncovering what clinicians of the past experienced.

Biography has recently become especially interesting for two reasons. One is that some scholars have turned away from grand historical narratives, and biography offers them a way of retaining narrative without taking responsibility for explicit generalizing beyond an individual life. The second reason is that, as in medical education, cases do teach. One can learn about what was going on in medicine in any time and place through the specifics of a life. What was it like to practice in *x* place in *y* years? What was the common experience in a laboratory in *x* century in *y* country? To what extent did doctors in *x* have to get along with other healers in the same time and place – and how well did they all carry it off? Indeed, any "microhistory" can serve to bring distant time near so that one can examine general points more closely.

Particularly interesting in recent medical history are accounts of healers' work that reveal how they interacted with their patients as well as their colleagues. One historian, Michael MacDonald, has worked through the detailed notes of a seventeenth-century physician in Buckinghamshire.[8] Another, Laurel Thatcher Ulrich, has published an account based on the diary of a midwife/healer in late-eighteenth-to-early-nineteenth-century Maine.[9] Both accounts are very rich indeed. Broader samples of records of many healers' work turn up any number of patterns. Not least of those patterns: in the eighteenth and nineteenth centuries, physicians, at least, spent an enormous amount of energy trying to get patients to pay the fees for which they had been billed.

Another approach to understanding the healers of the past is to examine the ways in which groups of them functioned. Collective accounts of physicians or nurses in one area in one time period – even if they were not formally organized or even networked – have produced enlightening detail about those healers, whether of Amsterdam or Buenos Aires. We have accounts of women in colonial New England who, rather than physicians, until the late eighteenth century could be the first resort of most people in the community. We have accounts of practitioners and their practices both in eighteenth- and nineteenth-century Germany and in many areas of the UK and localities in North America and Australasia. We have a complete and rich inventory of all of the physicians who ever practiced in Norway. Where groups of practitioners did form an organization, again historians have often unearthed at least the formal aspects of their existence. The history of professional associations is very rich – and very revealing (as I note again below, in discussing social institutions).

Both individual lives and the "biographies" of groups and institutions have inherent drama, even suspense, as in any good story. But beyond narrative and biography, historians have raised the question of how healers saw themselves – and of how they tried to project this self-image in the public realm. Healing may have been private, but the identity of the healer was a social phenomenon. Physicians in the eighteenth-century marketplaces could display their instruments or other symbols of professional competence to claim a social identity. In the fifteenth century, the physician could wear a distinctive long robe, in the twentieth a white lab coat. In 1914, a British surgeon, Harry Platt, who had been visiting the United States, returned home and explicitly urged his colleagues to adopt the wearing of the white coat to claim status by reminding patients and the public that doctors represented science. As long ago as 1930, the American historian Richard Shryock wrote a history of the "Public Relations of the Medical Profession," and others have followed in his footsteps.[10]

Heroic Figures

Historians may therefore write about the changing "image" of the physician and about specific healers of the past. Implicit in such material is a major function of the history of medicine: to set up models for current healers of all kinds. Like it or not, portraits of the great persist and can be understood as heroic narratives: not only those from the classical period, but Giovanni Morgagni, whose late eighteenth-century work set the stage for systematic pathology; Florence Nightingale, the putative founder of nursing; Robert Koch, who did so much to show a bacterial basis for many diseases; Ronald Ross, who in the 1890s convincingly established the mosquito vector for malaria; Santiago Ramón y Cajal, who advanced the neurone theory; Helen Taussig, who introduced the "blue baby operation"; Elizabeth Kenny, who revolutionized the treatment of polio. The list goes on and on.

In 1892, at a celebration of Louis Pasteur's seventieth birthday, Joseph Lister gave the chief address, and afterward Pasteur rose and embraced him. Everyone present understood the symbolism: they were two great figures who, despite much opposition, initiated a new era in medical theory and practice. Even today, most educated people from Western and non-Western cultures will recognize these heroes.

Heroes and heroines of course had failings, and historians have often pointed out such shortcomings. Many important overachievers, for example, showed a tendency to self promotion. Some, however accomplished, were brutal with patients or ruthless with colleagues or students. A young American physician in Paris, who greatly admired Guillaume Dupuytren's work and teaching in surgical pathology, nevertheless reported disapprovingly in 1833, "If his orders are not immediately obeyed he thinks nothing of striking his patient or abusing him most harshly. A very favorite practice of his during his consultations is to make a handle of the noses of his patients . . . with any disease of the head."

Yet in finding positive models, medical historians can focus on some contributions of a healer who might be worth examining. An ideal physician, in particular, may embody penetrating intelligence, plus feminine or masculine or human ideals of care, of learning, of leading, and of selflessness that can inspire, not only practitioners and students preparing for a career in health care, but all of those touched by the positive aspects of medicalization.

The Sick Person

In addition to the drama of the healer, there was a second drama. What happened to the person who became sick, who got well, or who died? Or what happened to someone who lived a long time with a chronic condition? The latter is a particular concern of modern historians who have to deal with aging populations.

A Person Suffering Illness

Healers were of course supposed to heal the sick. But as the process of medicalization proceeded, just who was sick became problematic. Some historians tried to follow sociologists' distinction between disease, which observers – especially physicians – could detect in a person, and illness, which was based on the perceptions and feelings of the person.

Historians have in fact drawn on accounts recorded by patients, on the one hand, and also, on the other hand, on eyewitness reports of disease processes taking place in people and the reactions of those people. The eyewitnesses were of course usually doctors. Regardless of source, the story of the life of every ailing person carried in it the potential for drama. A large number of patients' stories, taken together, make for

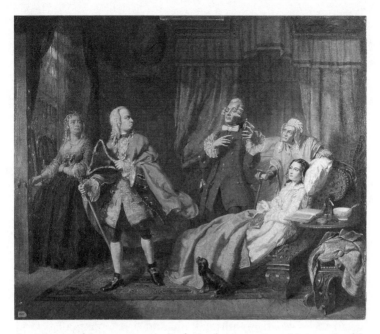

A patient making a consumer's choice between practitioners, in this case rejecting the English physician, Oliver Goldsmith (1728–1774, who was also, incidentally, a famous literary figure) in favor of treatment by an apothecary.

Source: Oil painting by Thomas Hall, Wellcome Library, London. Courtesy of the Wellcome Trust Medical Photographic Library.

grand drama, as in an epidemic or the account of a particular affliction suffered by many people.

Before the middle of the twentieth century, physicians' accounts constituted the core sources for medical history. Since that time, however, historians have ever more frequently sought patients' own stories as well as the testimonies of non-physician healers. Patient accounts not only enrich the narratives of medical history but are also absolutely essential to the narratives written about humble folk, "from the bottom up."

An abundance of source material from people's accounts of their ailments and illnesses has survived from most historical eras. They have left diaries and journals, autobiographical accounts, and letters. Some patients even in good health detailed every twinge and fear. Robert Hooke, the notable early modern scientist, on November 22 in 1673 wrote in his diary, "Slept very little all night, I suppose twas the heat of the fire and partly Coffe, the powder of which I fear lay in my Stomack and did me much harm . . . First began to leave off my physick ale and drink plain ale – God succeed it." Or on May 6, 1676: "very much out of order. Ulcer in nose. Sick in stomach. Cordiall made me worse. Vomited with whale bone a little." But all of the time Hooke was carrying on his usual activities. Or we know from Samuel Pepys' famous seventeenth-century diary that he caught a cold 102 different times in a ten-year period.

Sufferers' testimonies also contain often-vivid accounts of encounters with healers as well as the effects of each and every treatment, with details about how particular potions affected the course of the illness or the general health of the writer. Indeed, some such journals and letters tend to be day-by-day lists of miseries with the usually inevitable failure of "cures." The poet Samuel Coleridge in 1813 wrote in a letter of his encounter with self dosing with violent purgatives:

> I sent for 5 grains of Calomel & 15 of Jalap – & I cannot but suspect, that some carelessness was used in weighing the former, and a much larger dose sent – for all the next Day . . . I was alternately sick and griped to a degree, I had never before any conception [of]. – The pain & still more the state of my skull benumbed & stupefied, by the violent strainings,

alarmed me: & even yesterday I could retain nothing on my Stomach till late evening. This day I am much recovered; but still unable to sit down to the dinner-table.

Curiously, it has been customary for patients to make sense of what is happening by establishing a rational narrative. Something happened, and the illness followed. Recovery could follow as another chapter in the narrative. Usually a sequence of events suggested that one event caused the next one. Eventually this narrative custom in sickness reflected (and may have been encouraged by) the familiar case history from medical literature, an aspect of medicalization, as some scholars have pointed out. And where the thoughts and feelings of the ill person were included, the case could take on a literary appeal (which, as an "insider's" viewpoint, can define the category of biography). But such "inside" accounts could tend to be so idiosyncratic that they are not necessarily helpful to the historian.

The category of biography that is so conspicuous in histories of medical practitioners has not been as frequently used in the case of patients or sick people, except in some extraordinary accounts of people who suffered attacks of mental illnesses. To be the subject of biographical interest, one has to have some qualification other than being afflicted by a disease. The illnesses of kings, generals, presidents, saints, artists, and writers are of interest because of some other attribute of the sick person. Some, like polio victim President Franklin Roosevelt, qualify because they heroically overcame their disabilities. But there has not been much audience for extended accounts of what it was like to be miserable and sick. Or, like most people who cared little for cleanliness before sanitation, to suffer from "the itch." There continue to be far more biographies or autobiographies of caregivers than of those being cared for.

Moreover, as historian Anne Digby observes, patient accounts, in addition to being fragmentary, have caused other problems: "recorded lay perceptions and experiences of sickness are legion. But uneven coverage amongst different social groups has left the top and bottom of the social hierarchy much better served than those of the middling groups."[1]

Most of the best-known accounts of health and ill health, such as those of Dr Johnson and his associates, come from aristocrats and literate people in society. We know every detail of the physical presentations of Louis XIV. His physicians kept a journal for many years, recording not only every sign and symptom he experienced but each and every one of 2,000 or more occasions when doses and treatments were administered to make his digestive tract work rapidly – along with careful and devoted tabulations and descriptions of the resulting bowel movements. Similarly, there are the many accounts about people who were the objects of charity or those who appear in institutional records. All of this is rich, sometimes colorful material. But trying to figure out how typical or significant was any case or series of cases has created much contention among scholars.

Exactly what any patient or group of patients was experiencing is another problem that historians of medicine have addressed. In the traditional ceremony of diagnosing the patient, physicians long made a distinction between signs and symptoms, a distinction that somewhat paralleled that between disease and illness. Signs were what were observable – a flushed face, a thready pulse, convulsions, weight loss. Symptoms were what the patient felt and reported, such as pains, nausea, or dizziness. Obviously in infants most diagnosis was based on signs, and only older children could begin to contribute symptoms – what they were experiencing. An account of the onset and course of the illness – "the history," which helped greatly in diagnosis – could of course come from either the patient or family and friends.

The problem was that many conditions were not clear-cut or consistent. For generations, as medical historians have pointed out, in the West, masturbation was considered an illness, and historians have had a lot of fun ridiculing ways in which that and various other sexual functions and malfunctions were medicalized. For a very long time, "fever" was a disease. Later, it was a symptom. Or, to cite another kind of example, this one from the anthropologists, in one Native American group, the Papago, obesity was considered a normal condition, and parents would bring into the clinic for diagnosis an "ill" child whom most of the rest of the world would have considered healthfully trim. In short, personal and social perceptions as well as subjective feelings could define whether or not one was sick.

The Sick Role

For a long time, historians and social scientists showed that illnesses could have social components. And yet everyone knew that "being sick" was a major human concern and experience. As Molière in 1659 had his rascally quack doctor say, "Hippocrates says, and Galen by undoubtful arguments demonstrates, that a person is not in good health when he is ill."

In 1951, a sociologist, Talcott Parsons, took a major step in clarifying just what being a patient was all about. Medical historians have ever since drawn on Parsons and his later critics to understand what was happening in the past as well as in the mid-twentieth century and after. What Parsons did was to describe the "sick role." The culture made this role available, wrote Parsons, and cultural forces directed the "sick" person into a relationship with a healer so that the sick person could be relieved of the sick role.[2]

Being sick was socially deviant, in the Parsonian formulation. People who were voluntarily deviant, that is, who deliberately broke cultural standards, were criminals. But people who became deviant involuntarily took the sick role. In both cases, there were social forces that operated so that the person would be integrated back into society by correction or by cure. (Social forces could of course change the status of a syndrome. Alcoholism or homosexuality could be medical, or, at another time, demedicalized into some other category such as personal choice of lifestyle.)

The sick role had four aspects. First, the person was exempted from normal responsibility. Second, the person was not held to be responsible for the sickness and could not recover by his or her own free will. Third, the person had to see that sickness was an undesirable state and should wish to recover. And, fourth, the person was obliged to cooperate with "the treatment agent" so as to become non-deviant.

Historians, anthropologists, and sociologists all immediately found problems in the idea of the sick role – at the same time as they found the general concept of the sick role useful for understanding what it meant to be a patient in any society. A deviant person – including a sick person – threatened social stability because that person was not playing his or her proper, assigned social role.

Too many sick people could threaten the whole social structure (one would think immediately of the HIV/AIDS crisis threatening to destroy social functioning in parts of Africa at the beginning of the twenty-first century, if not the destruction of Native American societies by new diseases brought them by explorers and colonists after 1492).

Some physically deviant people, such as albinos, could be made into social totems (in classical times, as I have noted, epilepsy was the divine illness) – but they still suffered segregation. Members of communities have also often resisted supporting people excused from ordinary responsibilities. And should one interfere if the gods were using a disease to punish someone? Such a question was raised when inoculation against smallpox came into the West in the early eighteenth century.

But to what extent must a person in a culture conform to that culture? This is an eternal human question. As historians of disability point out, people with physical "handicaps" such as missing limbs could be marginalized in society by being labeled sick. Some historians have characterized reintegrating the patient as a way of keeping order in society. Or scholars have cited a long record of cases in which governments have declared non-conformist enemies to be "sick" – at one point, vocal political resisters in the old Soviet Union and hippies in the USA. In 1930s Brazil, authorities utilized medical personnel and facilities to combat, by "curing," an Afro-Brazilian religious movement that involved spirit possession.

Looking at health and healing in terms of a deviant sick role permits many scholars to criticize attempts to make sick people better. They note that medicalization may not always have been desirable, much less necessary. Correcting left-handedness in children – for generations in parts of the West a presumably undesirable deviant condition – provides an instructive example. Another example sure to instigate heated discussions even among scholars is circumcisions of various kinds that have had medical rationales. Moreover, historians can point out that vendors of profitable medicines, from early quacks to modern pharmaceutical corporations, certainly had an interest in seeing more people labeled sick. Of great interest, for instance, are those vendors who sold cures to women for various "female troubles" that may or may not have constituted an illness in earlier or later times.

Or, by assuming that the professional experts were neutral, agents of medicalization could further various social agendas, whether political or moral. There are numerous historical examples. What drugs should be controlled or forbidden? What sexual behaviors? Are beggars sick? And, in addition, labeling someone sick introduces the opportunity for powerful technological interventions in the name of medicine, such as drugging, surgery, or genetic alteration, many of which may be irreversible. Historians find themselves caught up in such controversial viewpoints from both past and present.

Focusing on the Individual

Above all, the sick role permits, in the name of health, making social improvement focus on the individual and his or her healing expert, as historians are busy pointing out. In the early twentieth century, when the germ theory was having a maximum effect on public health efforts, the problem of tuberculosis was most often met, not by correcting the physical and social conditions in which the pathogenic bacteria thrived, but by isolating each individual patient (to prevent contagion) and treating him or her. And this same model was often followed in campaigns to contain sexually transmitted diseases, tracking down specific agents of infection and trying to treat and isolate each of these infected persons, rather than making fundamental behavioral or social changes. In industry, when a worker fell ill from silicosis or metal dust poisoning or some other industrial disease, the treatment was to discharge the individual, not to improve the working conditions.

It is easy to see, therefore, that historians have had much opportunity to demonstrate that casting people in the sick role, and turning all problems into individual rather than social problems, shows that medicalization had powerful conservative aspects, for no social change was required when a social problem became a sickness to be cured on an individual basis. The only problem to worry about, then, as historians have pointed out, was how to pay for the individual professional healer.

At the same time, the sick role permitted another cultural trend to flourish over many ages: the philanthropic impulse to help by healing, referred to above, in the healing drama. A number of scholars have outraged colleagues by suggesting that genuine, warm, humanitarian impulses to cure the sick were but unintended ways of exploiting one's fellow humans for gain. Other historians have written about the charitable impulse itself and the ways in which kindly people have been able to help those who were unhappy in the sick role. Human wisdom tells us that, yes, some people liked being ill, but others did not.

People who are cast in a sick role, by themselves or others, clearly are out of adjustment with the local culture. But there are and were ways of being deviant other than in social functioning. What if one needed to get right with God or the gods? In the eighteenth century in India, smallpox had its own deity, called Sitala in northern India. Inoculation, carried out by a special group of "mark-makers," was a form of worship or propitiation of this goddess.

Indeed, through much of the history of medicine, people assumed that supernatural forces were causing physical problems, usually as punishment for breaking taboos or for other kinds of individual and collective sins. Historians have taken pains to try to understand how people at different times believed that God had sent a plague or an individual illness as a punishment. Such faithful people often tied medicine to morals or morals to medicine. In the Old Testament, God repeatedly punished groups of people with pestilence along with famine and war. Job suffered any number of painful symptoms. Psalm 38 specifies that "There is no health in my whole frame because of my sin." While sickness reminded one of one's misdeeds, of course hope for recovery made one think of salvation.

Historians have in fact recently taken great interest in exploring the relationship between religion and medicine in many societies. Was Christianity or Hinduism or Shintoism at any stage compatible with medicine? How much did the religion and medicine have in common, and to what extent did tension and conflict develop? Or, famously, did John Wesley, the founder of Methodism, damage his religious mission or facilitate it by writing a popular book of medical advice for ordinary people?

Much more central to medical history, however, is the drama of the patient who, regardless of social circumstance, had to get herself or himself right with nature. Or perhaps it was the same thing as religion. In standard theologies, after all, nature embodied the will of the Almighty. Lester King writes of the Galenic tradition, " 'according to nature' meant something both prevalent and desirable. 'Contrary to nature' was abnormal and undesirable. The natural implied a standard to which things ought to conform."[3] King quotes Daniel Sennert from the seventeenth century, who, in words that a later sociologist might have used, observed, "All men consider themselves healthy when, through the help of bodily parts, they are able to perform the functions according to nature, and necessary for life, without impairment (*vitio*) or hindrance . . . Persons are considered sick who cannot perform those activities, or at least, not without impairment."

So far historians have identified one major change in the meaning of what was wrong with a patient who in one sense or another was at variance with nature. Most medical and health experts of the early nineteenth century continued to assume that disease was an unnatural condition. Physicians attempted to get the patient back into harmony with nature. By the late nineteenth century, particularly after the introduction of technological aids such as the clinical thermometer and sphygmomanometer (to measure blood pressure), experts conceptualized sickness as abnormality – deviance from the normal. Disease became a state of a person's body, not an independent entity. And medical historians, too, have been caught up in the tension between believing abnormality a specific condition, on the one hand, and on the other believing it just a variation on the normal bell curve that entered general thinking by the early twentieth century to conceptualize differences in height or intelligence.

One subject from the middle of the natural–normal–deviant controversy in the late nineteenth century that has attracted the attention of historians has been the idea of degeneracy. Degeneracy was a hereditary process that typically intensified through generations. A degenerate human being presumably reversed the process of evolution, or simply exemplified or extended human blight. People with epilepsy or mental illness or any number of physical problems could be classified as biologically deteriorated. So could people manifesting deviant behavior (especially alcoholism). In addition, whole "races" of people had their "otherness" biologized. The roots of the idea of degeneracy and the ways in which it played out, especially in mental illnesses, has consti tuted a particularly fertile field for historical investigation.

One of the controversies that emerged out of nineteenth-century "degeneracy" had special reverberations at the turn of the twenty-first century: the notion of inherited or constitutional diseases, an idea that flourished before and after degeneracy. When disease was a vague entity, people had predispositions or peculiar susceptibilities to various complaints. Illnesses occurred because of one's constitution ("constitutional weakness" or even "constitutional distemper"). But not always. And so individual susceptibilities and immunities softened to become mere tendencies. But at the same time, those weaknesses or vulnerabilities became part of one's person.

After scientists adopted Mendelian genetics based on immutable inherited traits, beginning in 1900, a disease could become an inherited "trait." Investigators immediately identified specific diseases, most famously Huntington's disease (a degenerative brain disorder), that followed Mendelian laws of inheritance. Then for decades, beginning in 1959, convincing evidence became available that chromosomal configurations lay behind some mental retardation, sickle-cell anemia, cystic fibrosis, and other disorders. And historians are having a field day trying to sort out different ways in which people of the past conceptualized not only illness but an individual person's illnesses and susceptibilities. In recent times, there has tended to be a view that one might be just a part of a "population at risk" for some disorder or another. The tension has become acute between social imperatives, the idea that disease may be an attribute of a population, and individual recognition, often conceptualized as recognition of one's own body. Historians with political-moral interests are in their element with such historical material, as I comment again below in connection with social ethics.

The Physical Self

One major way of understanding a thing is to know what it is not. And so it was with an individual's being ill. In a traditional formulation, Galen held that health and disease were opposites, so that if it was possible to establish one, the other would be clear. Therefore to write about the experience of a sick person, a historian has to suggest what a healthy person was, in any particular historical context.

Most ideas about sick people referred more directly to the ways in which the individual was deviating from being his or her natural self. Or from some ideal of the self. Historians have followed the idea of deviating from one's self in two major directions. First, they have explored how the physical self was the point of comparison, how people thought of their physical selves in such a way that they understood being in a state of sickness to be different from the way in which the physical self usually operated (as did Sennert, who was just quoted). Second, scholars have followed ideas about "the body" into many aspects of health and illness. Each of these ideas about how the self was normal and natural (as opposed to requiring a sick role) has attracted any number of scholars and has led them sometimes far afield. "The body," writes Linda Hogle, "is an object of renewed interest in the social sciences. Yet theories of the body's relationship to self and society are polarized between an unproblematized view of biology without context and a view that reduces the body to little more than language and representation."[4]

One set of ideas about the healthy body came directly from ideas put forth by medical writers. Indeed, the attractiveness of each of the changing medical models of somatic, or bodily, functioning was one of the most powerful forces making for medicalization of the broader society throughout Western history, and the same can be said of medical traditions in other parts of the world. What the doctors and allied biomedical scientists thought continued to reverberate throughout the rest of each society even as the ideas changed – and where culture helped shape medical thinking. Something as apparently straightforward as anatomy, for example, was deeply influenced by religious ideas in different times and places.

The major model that lasted the longest in the West – from ancient Greek times to almost the nineteenth century – was that of the four humors. When blood, black bile, yellow bile, and phlegm were in balance in a person's body, the person was healthy. As Hippocrates observed, "It seems to me . . . necessary to know which of man's diseases arise from the *powers*, and which from the *structures* . . . By powers I mean the intensity and strength of the humours, and by structures the conformations of the body."

Embedded in humoral thinking was the idea that an internal homeostasis, or balance, constituted health. Too much or too little of any of the humors constituted sickness. Scholars have examined all of the humors and humoral deviations and are always finding new aspects of them. Currently medievalists are taking special interest in how the general idea of "plethora," in the form of too much blood, came into being, and how plethora would call for treatment by bleeding.

The age of reason brought forth many ideas, not only of pathology but of healthy functioning of the body. Was the stomach a chemical cauldron or a grinding machine? What was the material basis for the nervous system? Deviating from healthy functioning – whatever it was – would establish in an individual a state, and role, of sickness. Scholars have devoted much effort to attempting to reconstruct not only technical but popular versions of the theoretical and technical discourses about the human body before, during, and after the early modern period. And they have found, for example, that as eighteenth-century investigators established local sites of diseases (anatomical pathology), so the basis for healthy functioning tended to appear to medical thinkers to be both physical in nature and localized in the body. Breathing obviously required lungs that worked.

Systems and Organs

Eventually educated people began to speak rather generally about "the system" operating in each person's body. Again, historians have uncovered a variety of versions of this idea that were both technical and popular. By the early nineteenth century, the system was based on the idea of organs, each of which served some purpose. Of course with various thinkers and various individuals, the array of organs could vary. Scholars have worked to make sense of past thinkers' teleologies of organs and the system (that is, the purpose and useful function of each one – satirized in the answer to the question of why the Almighty created us with noses: obviously to hold our spectacles). Many early nineteenth-century thinkers, for example, adopted the thinking of phrenologists, who believed that in the brain resided organs of various personality traits, such as "amativeness." They even posited an organ of murder. But the idea of a general system, functioning as God or nature designed it, survived along with thinking in terms of organs. In 1868, the French neurologist J. M. Charcot told his students, "Symptoms ... are in reality nothing but the cry from suffering organs." Even today, a historian can point out, it is still possible to speak not only of the kidneys or heart but of a nervous system or of disorders of one's gastrointestinal system.

During the nineteenth century, two things happened in the West. First, physicians began to specialize in the disorders of one organ or system. Even on the popular level, patent medicine cures typically targeted a particular organ or system, as in Sanford's Liver Invigorator or Fendt's Bronchial Cigarettes.

And, second, the new mechanical age provided other types of elements in terms of which people could conceptualize their bodies. The body could be a steam engine, and, in popular treatises, children were urged to eat heartily, just as one would shovel coal into a steam locomotive so that it could burn the fuel to make energy. The nervous system became first a telegraph system and then a telephone system with a central exchange: sensory messages came in, and motor responses went out to move the limbs or whatever. Scholars continue to point out the consequences as such metaphors came to be taken surprisingly seriously (the nervous impulse does not, in fact, always behave like an electrical communication).

At the end of the nineteenth century, information about bodily processes and disease processes had accumulated so that still another model of the body began to crystallize. First, investigators noticed that bodies differed. Some bodies would harbor dangerous microbes but not succumb to a dangerous reaction. Other bodies would develop the expected disease so that the body would become an obvious clinical "case." Then people began focusing on independent elements in the body, not only cells to battle bacteria, but a variety of complex chemicals and, eventually, particularly when people were aware of AIDS at the end of the twentieth century, "the immune system." The immune system could react to "foreign" invaders and substances. In the one case, fighting germs and chemicals, the immune system preserved health. But immune reactions could also cause sickness. The term "allergy" entered medicine in 1906.

Eventually, one no longer spoke of one's healthy body, but of one's healthy immune system. As early as the 1990s, anthropologist Emily Martin even detected an "immune machismo," quoting a young male medical resident who "claimed that his immune system could 'kick ass.'"[5] He expressed a medicalized idea, but also one obviously influenced by a culture in which people were blamed for being sick or poor or otherwise weak – just as, in an earlier age, people believed that women's bodies, dominated by reproductive organs, made them emotional and passive.

By the early twentieth century, the idea of the human body was extremely complicated, but, as historians point out, there continued both in technical Western physiology and in popular thinking the idea of a balance or homeostasis. One new element at the time was the idea of deficiency diseases. What if something necessary for health was missing? Shortages of endocrine products (including thyroid secretions and insulin) or the newly discovered vitamins could easily push people into the sick role. So, too, could excesses – as of stomach acids or adrenal products.

Scholars who have made much of technical ideas of the body and popularization of those ideas have only begun to explore new ways of thinking that came in the late twentieth century. Tracing the origins of such thinking continues. In the 1970s, many biomedical thinkers put a great emphasis on environment – people thought that water and air and other ambient forces had decisive effects on a body constantly adapting to the environment. But then so did Hippocrates. And later, with the rise of a dream of genetic engineering and concern about individual susceptibilities, all of the previous ideas could be read as existing in special combination so that each body was special and distinctive.

It was in the face of such material that a whole generation of scholars, many of them historians, began to write about past ideas of the body. Medicine in general had a long tradition of physicians' using their knowledge about the body to establish their authority. Physicians had a special qualification because they knew anatomy from dissecting cadavers. As early as the fourteenth century, medicalization had proceeded sufficiently that educated people thought of the heart as a literal thing rather than something metaphorical or an occult symbol. This tradition of anatomizing, and physicians' role in death, when the body turns into a cadaver, put physicians into a special relationship with "the body," a charged and even mystical relationship that historians are still exploring.

Social Meanings of "The Body"

But some recent scholars have gone further in asserting that the body was not just a physical object. They can track this idea directly to the philosopher René Descartes, who in the seventeenth century insisted on separate realms for the mind/soul and the body. The body therefore came to have a different meaning for modern people than it did in ancient and medieval times. Then in the third quarter of the twentieth century, Michel Foucault was especially influential in suggesting that a body could be a sociocultural construct, indeed, an object and instrument of political power. He went on to suggest how a state, for example, could claim control over a person's body or how a local establishment could indirectly affect and direct a self as well as the body in which the self resided – even while appearing to let the person control his or her self.

It is easy to see that this sense that each person's body is special raised the consciousness of scholars about ways in which conceptions of physical/mental bodies had in the past led to individual and group misunderstanding, injustice, and discrimination. At those times, the specialness of individual bodies permitted those bodies to be grouped with others in inappropriate ways, such as "race" and gender or generic "other." Historians therefore are still exploring how healers, political authorities, and cultural authorities all attempted to control various bodies at different times. A whole literature appeared on "the colonized body" as an aspect of imperialism.

If the social role of an individual was tied to his or her body, the experts on the body were still the physicians, whether acting as life insurance examiners or as providers of knowledge about anatomy, physiology, and pathology. And that medical knowledge, some scholars have pointed out, could assist sociopolitical authorities in controlling other people's bodies. The paradigm case was of course the way in which female bodies had been controlled in male-dominated societies.

Feminist theorists and women's historians eventually began to reconceptualize the ways in which gender had always been a part of ideas about the body – mostly, these scholars pointed out, men's ideas. Women's historians therefore added a new dimension to medical history, drawing as well on other currents that remain remarkably stimulating and productive of new scholarship. How big should one's body be? How should it be decorated and clothed, that is, how should the body be extended? Are glasses, hearing aids, canes, and wheelchairs not part of one's body? On another level, what is the inner structure of the body and what are its boundaries? And, again, how does it function? What about body gestures?

"The body" has therefore in such ways taken on multifarious and changing meanings. Scholars now exhume sources from which one can learn how women and men thought about their own bodies – their selves. In the early nineteenth century, patients sent to Samuel Hahnemann, the founder of homeopathy, excruciatingly detailed accounts of the ways in which they worried about their bodies and asked for appropriate medications. They could report moods and a general sense of weakness. They could imagine what was happening to their organs and fluids. One, who would report even a minor "discomfort in tip of nose," recorded for just one day: "Before breakfast, pressure in stomach area as if there was a stone lying inside . . . Tingling at several points on body. One cough. Pressure in side. Discomfort in anus. Feeling of having a cold. Pain in both temples." Martin Dinges points out how such material shows the many ways in which patients, over time, perceived their bodies and communicated with physicians about those bodies.[6] In early modern times, sickness was personal and internal. By the late nineteenth century, one could experience standard germs invading one's body.

Always, of course, it was physicians who had written most not only about systems and the body, but about separate parts of the body such as the foot or the pudenda. If one removed the (male) physician from the narrative (except as, sometimes, a historical source), a new kind of history of medicine and health could, and did, develop.

Moreover, it was a segment of medical history that moved smoothly across boundaries. To recover the ways in which people experienced their bodies, one could turn not only to personal accounts but to many sources, such as art or politics (at the turn of the eighteenth century, social commentators could refer to "an ulcer in the body politic"). By pursuing the body in health and disease, medical historians therefore could find themselves drawn deeply into many other fields of history, particularly virtually every type of social history. Did one count "bodies"? One was into demography. Did a scholar examine the body as a basis for social classification? Not only dwarfs and the disabled but, again, the whole concept of "race," and sometimes class, emerged. Did one work with the way in which people experienced their bodies? One could see that around 1800, for example, educated people believed that both body appearance and body movement expressed a person's soul. Later historians quickly found themselves trying to reconstruct versions of a social unconscious on the basis of experiencing one's body.

Women's historians were particularly effective in questioning the ways in which women of the past experienced their own bodies. Was a woman's self supposed to fit the physicians' portrayal of her body at a particular time? To what extent could one separate health from the body? And then these questions were applied also to men, to all people. One particularly productive strand lay in the history of madness – alienation from one's (embodied) self, but also, it turned out, alienation from society.

A great deal of what started out as histories of ideas of illness and health thus ended up as histories of ideas about the self (although the concept of self did not necessarily work in non-Western societies). Changing general ideas provided one set of narratives, as "the body" was transformed into "the self" and the culturally "other," and scholars from different fields such as literature were drawn into source material originally claimed for historians of medicine. Accounts of people's bodies, and the selves associated with those bodies, tended to become narratives, narratives of who a person was. "Insider" stories had a texture that could give the illusion of "experience." By adding a time element – the "story" of the self – scholars could shift their focus from lasting general facts about the self to an individual's personal feelings. Information about the lives of patients thus took on new meanings for health, illness, and disability.

Such explorations apply only to those patients whose illnesses were drawn out so that there was more to an illness, and to the personal and social reactions to that illness, than just some symptoms that were resolved quickly either fatally or favorably before any negotiated social role could develop. The sick role was made for lingering or chronic more than acute disease. The person who was struck with violent stomach cramps, nausea, diarrhea, and fever with delirium, and who expired within two days – as did a substantial part of the human race – did not have time to develop much narrative or to "experience" the illness.

The Autonomy of Patients

Hidden in the contemporary social scientists' theories and in the bottom-up, subjective histories of the disease experience of ordinary people was a major issue: how much agency (the ability of a person to make choices for himself or herself) did a patient, forced into a sick role, have? It turned out that patients never entrusted their bodies entirely to physicians. Late twentieth-century social scientists, on their part, had found that, especially in chronic diseases, all aspects of the sick role were being negotiated as patients had to deal not only with doctors but with medical institutions, such as hospitals and aftercare, in which status and even basic identity could become major issues for a patient. The longer a sickness lasted, the more likely was the patient to negotiate and renegotiate the sick role and the social terms in which that role was played out. Indeed, the ways in which patients from the beginning of history manipulated their health care systems was a drama in itself.

Once having introduced the power of the physician and his or her institutions, such as hospitals, in the past, scholars now looked in greater detail at the course of the patient's relationship to the doctor in individual cases in different time periods. Historians found, of course, that patients had always had independence and agency in their relationships with healers and healing institutions. In the eighteenth century, the physician to the impetuous Richard Nash, a notable public figure in Bath, at one point asked Nash if he had followed the physician's prescription. "Egad, if I had," expostulated Nash, "I should have broke my neck, for I flung it out of the window."

Investigators have found that in past times, sick people from humble walks of life, as well as the well educated, exercised their independence in many ways. For one thing, they could choose not to have medical advice. Or they could choose to consult irregular or quack practitioners, or to employ folk remedies. Mary Lindemann has found a record from 1767 in which a patient ill with consumption (tuberculosis of the lungs), and seeking some effective course of medicine, consulted in turn a local hangman, a well-qualified physician, a cowherd in a nearby village, and then a physician in another town. And of course no one at the time thought that this sequence of seeking for a cure was unusual. People of that time were all, as Lindemann suggests, "medically promiscuous."[7]

Scholars have also uncovered the ways in which women as patients over the centuries sometimes used their conventional gender identity to manipulate the sick role and so exercise agency in a variety of ways. The female "nervous invalid" of the late nineteenth century has especially generated a large and lively series of interpretations.

The little dramas of ordinary people and oppressed groups who participated actively in fashioning and using their sick roles could add up to major dramas. Just at the end of the twentieth century, several strands came together into a major new type of history: disability history. The immediate cause was the remarkable shift in advanced economies from acute diseases to chronic diseases. People with both fatal and non-fatal chronic diseases had to address just what their social role would be. Many refused to accept the inactivating and marginalizing roles found in most societies for those who did not recover normality. At least within limited areas, the permanently sick gloried in what abilities and agency they did have. Where once, especially from medieval times, disability had been an object of charity, now such a condition involved "rights." Physicians and other representatives of society who tried to escape their responsibility for the incurable or the perpetually sick therefore found that rules long accepted had to be modified or changed to accommodate a major new social power group, the disabled, along with the chronically ill.

It also had not taken feminist theorists and women's historians long to figure out that women for centuries had been treated in the West as disabled people who could not fully participate in society. They were handicapped by their sex. (And of course the same went for those carrying other labels, especially "racial" designations.) Since physicians had, in various societies, been leaders in describing and justifying the handicapped label for women, some historians of women's health and illness came, as I noted above, to focus on the drama of female suffering and female resistance to establishment medicine.

In the nineteenth and twentieth centuries, historians have found, the growing effectiveness of medical technology made a major modification to the usual struggles of patients to maintain agency. Especially beginning with the introduction of surgical anesthesia from 1846, services that physicians could offer began to appear both more and more desirable and, at the same time, beyond the control of patients. With changed terms of negotiation, patients lost autonomy – a process that continues to demand historical exploration. As does the high value members of some Western social groups put on "taking control" of one's own health (to the point of making a "living will").

Yet other historical narratives have been constructed around what it meant for a patient to have agency. Some scholars continued to focus on the details of the patient–doctor interaction, particularly for those periods when medicine was very personal and, indeed, the authority of the healer came more from his or her wisdom and character than from science. Scholars tracing the history of medical ethics (currently a very active field, as I shall note again) have noticed that before the twentieth century, medical ethics involved mutual obligations – the duty of the patient to the physician as much as restraints on the physician. By the twentieth century, ethics were those applying to the conduct of health care personnel, to protect the patient from neglect or abuse in the health care system. Beginning in the 1970s, this relationship took on the appearance of customer protection – and the "patient" turned into a "consumer."

Stimulated by histories of modern consumer culture, there is now a whole field covering the history of the ill person as a consumer of health care products and services (not least the services of the physician "provider"). The consumer identity can be applied to patients in any age and most cultures. Historians of the late twentieth century have to contend with the actions of many patients who were very well-informed consumers in medical theories and therapies of their times. But this story is also part of a recent chapter in the traditional, fascinating history of popularization of ideas about health and illness, and particularly of self-treatment and across-the-counter medicines. As numerous historians have shown, self-doctoring could be very colorful, from patent medicine advertisements to do-it-yourself medical manuals, including the instructions of one early nineteenth-century author for amputating one's own leg.

Following the theme that sick people had agency and could make consumer choices, many historians have broadened the history of medicine to include all of the medical marketplace at any time (an appropriate development for an age in which so many opinion leaders praise "market forces"). Hence the history of family recipes for various ailments, of commercial preparations, and of the entire spectrum of "irregular" quacks and practitioners has (as noted above concerning healers) become mainstream medical history.

Historians of early modern Europe have been especially excited to be able to reconstruct the incredible range of choices – including the established medical hierarchy of physicians, surgeons, and apothecaries – open to consumers of healing services. Laurence Brockliss and Colin Jones use the aristocratic Madame de Sévigné of the late seventeenth century to show both the lack of distance between elite and non-elite healers in one household and Madame de Sévigné's shrewd consumerism. An apothecary and physician won her confidence because "they are the first to condemn their own remedies when they don't suit."[8]

Moreover, that same excitement has also passed to those working in the histories of developing countries, where "folk medicine" was particularly important in defining cultural as well as disease entities. It turns out that people's choosing one kind of health care or another, or more than one at a time, is dramatic on several levels – not least the heroic role of people in the past who in illness chose to ignore either widely sanctioned folk customs or regular or Western medicine in either alien or domestic guises.

Altogether, the ways in which patients reacted or did not react to their illnesses provided a gauge of the extent to which the processes of medicalization proceeded or receded over time. After the body became an object, it was easy in the West to medicalize birth, death, and the whole life cycle. Or, in any culture, how did patients use the alternatives available to them? Above all, how did they, as consumers, negotiate and renegotiate the sick role? Both individual and social answers provide powerful drama and continue to attract the excited (and often indignant) interest of medical historians. And of a lot of other people.

The Third Drama

Diseases

Beyond the doctor and the patient, there is another element in sickness, the disease. Indeed, most people would put the disease first. And certainly the struggle between humans and diseases makes for grand drama. Moreover, as each disease took on a separate identity in medical thinking, abstracted from many different personal experiences, the history of the disease created a drama of its own. How could that particular disease come to human beings? How did they deal with it?

A major disease was a major human problem, but apparently minor diseases, too, could have important consequences for individuals and societies. An everyday scratch could become infected. Subtle nutritional deficiencies, minor eye infections, and even colds (for example in an opera singer) could generate substantial social effects as well as personal disruption. In the late eighteenth century, Dominique-Jean Larrey, a French military surgeon, reported an attack of seasickness during an Atlantic storm: "The faculties of the mind suffer in common with the organs of animal life, and this change takes place to such a degree, that instead of dreading death, as in the commencement of the disease, their suffering is so intolerable that they desire it; and as I have seen, attempt to commit suicide."

What is a Disease?

As historians have investigated the specifics of the dramas of disease, they have run into a problem that has troubled physicians, scientists, philosophers, and other scholars: how does one know that a disease exists, and how does one know what the boundaries of any disease may be? The points of view range from commonsense observation of an ill person to a conviction that all diseases are social constructions, imagined entities invented by people with particular perspectives. Historians have found examples to illustrate the difficulties. Having wrinkles, for example, in the twentieth century could be a disease that required a highly trained medical person to perform "cosmetic" surgery to correct the condition. From a strictly social point of view, the ill person had to be restored to his or her social condition, what would be construed as normality – assuming that having smooth skin is normal. But many people would argue that wrinkles are not a disease. Or, if having wrinkles is a disease, how many wrinkles must one have to be sick? What is the threshold point at which a disease state exists?

By contrast, people who died of a dysentery or gangrene showed subjective and objective signs such that there could be no sensible way of denying that a sickness had struck them and that others undergoing similar experiences and showing similar signs probably were afflicted with the same kind of trouble. Some historians have written of disease that is an embodied experience (in the patient) or disembodied (generalized social experience that was given a name, like tonsillitis or a fractured skull).

Charles Rosenberg in a classic essay has shown that it is possible, without denying or minimizing the physical realities of disease processes, to recognize the social negotiation and filtering around disease entities that people in the past identified. He suggests that humans "frame" diseases in various configurations. Many scholars have worked with Rosenberg's metaphor or model to show how different societies over time created categories of sickness for healers, patients, and other cultural collaborators. Disease, Rosenberg writes, "is at once a biological event, a generation-specific repertoire of verbal

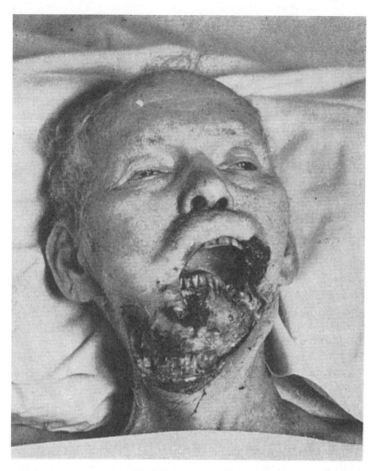

A patient with cancer of the jaw caused by smoking. This photograph is from the early twentieth century, just when, in industrialized countries, chronic illnesses like cancer and heart disease were becoming more prominent than acute infectious diseases.

Source: John Harvey Kellogg, *Tobaccoism, Or, How Tobacco Kills* (1923).

constructs reflecting medicine's intellectual and institutional history, an occasion for and potential legitimation of public policy, an aspect of social role and individual – intrapsychic – identity, a sanction for cultural values, and a structuring element in doctor–patient interactions." He goes on, "It is no accident that several generations of anthropologists have assiduously concerned themselves with disease concepts in non-Western cultures; for agreed-upon etiologies [causes] at once incorporate and sanction a society's fundamental ways of organizing its world."[1]

Simply by raising the question of changing definitions of diseases, Rosenberg shows how a whole program of historical inquiry is laid out. The concept of framing diseases embraces subjects and approaches from the broadest social questions to the most elemental intellectual and biological histories. Critics of Rosenberg's idea have argued that it assumes too much material reality in disease and not enough human agency in defining diseases. But in practice, Rosenberg's formulation accommodates most historians.

There are exceptional cases from the past that puzzle common sense – and medical historians. Such a case was that of Mary Mallon, known as "Typhoid Mary." A typhoid "carrier" in turn-of-the-century New York, every time she evaded the authorities and obtained a job as a cook, an outbreak of typhoid occurred where she worked. She was eventually interned and isolated permanently. As historian Robert Hudson asks: what does one do with Mary Mallon, "whose gallbladder teemed with typhoid bacilli" but caused Ms Mallon no symptoms at all?[2] She did not feel any illness, but to public health authorities and victims, she was diseased – and dangerous.

Most history does not turn on borderline or exceptional cases. We can usually trace how one set of observations was set forth by one observer – usually a physician reporting a limited number of cases. If other observers could also see what that observer saw, and could connect further, similar cases, then a disease, or at least a syndrome, came into the community (medical or lay or both). Reconstructing this tortured process of establishing and confirming the existence of a workable disease constitutes much good medical history. And when writers of the time followed a convention of science, they often added another historical dimension by naming the disease after the clinician who first saw a series of cases that were distinctively similar – Burkitt's lymphoma, for example, or Paget's disease or Pick's disease (there were two Picks, and one identified an edema and the other a brain syndrome, both named Pick's disease!). There are whole books listing medical conditions named after observant clinicians of the past. And of course history can be built into other diseases, which are named after places. Beyond calling syphilis the French disease or the Spanish disease in the sixteenth century, there were in the twentieth for example Murray Valley (Australia) encephalitis and Lyme (Connecticut) disease. And Lou Gehrig's disease (amyotropic lateral sclerosis or motor neurone disease) was actually named after a patient. Machado-Joseph disease is a type of cerebellar ataxia named after the two families in which the pattern of pathology was discovered.

The history of discovery, description, and definition of syndromes is one aspect of the history of disease. More broadly, the occurrence of an agreed-upon pattern of symptoms in numbers of people, over a period of time, is the basis for a large part of medical history. Thomas Sydenham, a justly famous English physician of the seventeenth century, put the matter simply: "Nature, in the production of disease, is uniform and consistent, so much so, that for the same disease in different persons the symptoms are for the most part the same, and the selfsame phenomena that you would observe in the sickness of a Socrates you would observe in the sickness of a simpleton."

Refining the Definitions

There are, as medical historians point out, the possibilities of perceiving any condition in a variety of ways. Cultural differences are endlessly fascinating. In one culture, a backache after physical exercise could be a sign that something was wrong. In another culture, the identical backache would be a sign that someone healthy had worked really hard. In Japan, one would not ordinarily go to a doctor because of suffering from the condition known as "hot flushes" or "hot flashes"; in the West, one might, for, by the late nineteenth century, menopause was being medicalized into a disease. And symptoms of apparently the same diseases can differ markedly from place to place as well as from time to time. In some groups in Africa, one type of bilharzia, a parasitic disease also known as schistosomiasis, generated complaints of abdominal pains, while Europeans suffering from what for some time was believed to be the same biological pathogen tended to focus on lassitude as the defining symptom. In mental diseases in the mid-twentieth century, people from some cultures tended to hear voices speaking to them in the second person, while patients in more developed countries tended to hear the voices using the third person. Or what in the West were emotional diseases, such as anxiety or depression, in some Asian cultures were experienced as physical, with digestive disorders and palpitations, for example.

To cite still another kind of example, what Westerners call cholera could be a named entity, "cholera." Or it could be vomiting-and-diarrhea disease, as some cultures called it, after the way in which it was experienced by the patient. Or, in different times and places, it could be described by symptoms, without a name that would give it a further identity. In each case, the history of that disease embodied a human problem that was, or could have been, general, but in each case the disease name gave it a slightly different place in the patient's social context.

Historians have also described how particular cultures and technologies changed the ways in which in any setting the people might define the illness they were seeing. A reading on a scale is the most obvious example, such as how much sugar was in the urine. Or a smear on the microscope slide. Perhaps the most notorious instance was determining exactly when a patient was suffering from some kind of poisoning – as opposed to carrying only a normal burden of the poisonous substance. In the late twentieth century, laboratory tests, not objective symptoms or the patient's sense of well-being, determined whether or not a person was showing the toxic effects of heavy metals, organic phosphates, or other chemicals. How technology came to triumph over clinical judgment (and sometimes did not!) has generated a number of historical accounts. Recent developments have brought more problems. Historians are trying to write about diseases that came to be conceived as operating in response to "risk factors." As the individual fell into statistical or genetic groups, he or she might fall victim to a condition for which he or she was at risk.

As health and health care became embedded in a highly complex and organized society, the demands of social organization, too, set up ways of defining disease. When life and health insurance developed in the late nineteenth century, physicians were pressed by responsible administrators to define whether or not a person had a particular disease – and in terms that could be generalized. The pressures of social organization were often successful in grouping symptoms into categories more meaningful for bureaucracies than for the patient and the physician. Of great social significance were those conditions for which a twentieth-century person could be certified to receive support because of disability. At one point in the United States, when polio would win a settlement but other conditions would not, compassionate physicians would label a Guillain-Barré syndrome "polio" to help the patient economically.

As use of efficient, standardized forms in either private practice or hospitals meant that patients had to be fitted into categories on the form, the rich clinical descriptions, in which the clinician could explore the individual complexity presenting before him or her, disappeared. Or people who ran hospitals had to decide how to classify patients. Before it was shown to be a vitamin deficiency, pellagra was frequently considered a mental disease because it often caused mental disturbances. The reclassification of people suffering from pellagra caused great political and administrative problems that historians have explored.

The difficulties of classification suffuse the historical record. Was a particular condition best categorized as an infectious disease? Should the patient be allowed an expensive medicine suitable only for acute fevers when he or she had a chronic fever? Or if a patient had particularly interesting symptoms, and if he or she fell into a specialist consultation, the specialist might well fix on the interesting tumor or infection and neglect the underlying or more general conditions existing in the patient, such as malnutrition. Indeed, many medical historians have made a special effort to show how current problems in medical practice had comparable – or identical – expressions in the past.

Paleopathology

Diseases have been with us always. Medical historians for a very long time have appropriated, or at least borrowed, the field of paleopathology. That is, how do we know that humans suffered from diseases before there were any written records? Is there some truth in the idea of a disease-free Garden of Eden at the beginning of human existence? The forthright answer is that evidence of disease processes has survived in human remains – mostly skeletons – from prehistoric people. Sometimes, of course, one can identify signs of violence, such as crushed skulls and decapitations. Much more interesting are characteristic signs of particular diseases such as tuberculosis of the bones or dietary insufficiency.

For the medical historian, paleopathology provides a powerful demonstration that disease is and has been a universal and constant experience of human beings. And yet anthropologists and paleopathologists have raised questions. Was it the development of agriculture and a sedentary group lifestyle that brought contagious diseases into prominence? How free of such diseases were the scattered hunter-gatherer societies? And, in the end, how much can one infer about patterns of incidence from paleopathological evidence?

In the closing years of the twentieth century, interest in paleopathology increased, and it continues. On the one hand, the discovery of the so-called Ice Man (whose 5,000-year-old remains were found in 1991 in ice in the mountains between Italy and Austria) and other preserved cadavers created much scientific as well as popular interest. From what illnesses or conditions did the Ice Man suffer? Were marks on his skin medical tattoos? On the other hand, technical means (most notably computerized tomography, or CT, scans and DNA fragment analysis) appeared that could greatly extend the ability of specialists in paleopathology to make diagnoses of diseases in people who died before written records. Evidence from Egyptian mummies was long of interest, but now it became possible to discern evidence not only of bone disease and tooth decay but of other ailments, including, for example, malaria and the common parasitic disease schisto-somiasis, associated with the Nile River. Or, to cite another example, mummies from the Andes show evidence of the same lymphotrophic retrovirus as is today found notably in Japan.

Particularly interesting evidence has also come from sampling human remains from historic periods, a way of checking on written records or filling in gaps. Most of this material has come from aggregating data from many graves. Thus investigators can show that women of the seventeenth century did indeed die very frequently in the course of childbirth and that during the harsh conditions of industri-alization in the nineteenth century, the nutritional status of ordinary people declined. Or such evidence can confirm that Native American populations suffered from many illnesses, particularly hemorrhagic diseases, even before Europeans introduced smallpox, influenza, and other virus diseases in the sixteenth century. Still unanswered – at least to many scholars' satisfaction – is whether or not paleopathology shows that lead poisoning (from wine in casks lined with metal or from lead conduits in the famous water system) was crucial in weakening the Roman Empire.

Epidemics

From the earliest historical records, it is clear that already in ancient times people identified patterns of illness and classi-fied them into disease entities that served for understanding and action (although historians continue to disagree about the appropriate translations in such documents). William H. McNeill, in his modern classic *Plagues and Peoples*, quotes a description from China in the first centuries AD: "Recently there have been persons suffering from epidemic sores which attack the head, face and trunk. In a short time, these sores spread all over the body. They have the appearance of hot boils containing some white matter. While some of these pustules are drying up, a fresh crop appears. If not treated early the patients usually die." The disease, McNeill concludes, must have been smallpox or measles.[3] But there will always be a scholar to disagree with him or with anyone else.

The most dramatic afflictions were of course what later became known as epidemic diseases, or, more generally, pestilences and plagues. While exactly what constituted the plague of the Philistines in the Old Testament is unknown, it is obvious that large numbers of people were suffering from similar symptoms. Much ink has also been spilled in attempts to identify the plague of Athens (430–427 BC) recorded by the historian Thucydides – was it anthrax, typhus, toxic shock syndrome? No one knows. Or the plague of Justinian that began in AD 541 and killed hundreds of thousands of people in Constantinople alone (there is now argument based on DNA evidence that the disease was indeed, as some historians claimed, bubonic plague).

In these instances of epidemics and in other occurrences of widespread suffering found in historical records, some distinctive disease spread rapidly and killed or incapacitated a notable number of people. In many cases, the record also suggests that the epidemic had powerful social effects, starting with battles lost and ramifying out into major social and economic consequences, including major demographic changes (see also below, the fifth drama). Exploring both the biological and social factors of each noticeable change in the health status of groups of people has kept historians busy for generations and has fueled many scholarly controversies. In colonial India, was the persistent toll of malaria, which depopulated whole villages, not more serious than recurrent waves of cholera? Historians combing evidence from the past continue to discover new episodes of epidemic disease, such as the smallpox pestilence of 1775–82 that swept all of North America, regardless of whether the local population was European or Native American.

Then scholars disagree concerning basic questions. How many people actually died? What effects did the experience have on survivors? What social institutions were changed? The great influenza pandemic of 1918–19 had few lasting effects on social institutions in many countries. Histories of that disease could therefore be largely colorful antiquarianism, or at the most demonstrations of beliefs at that time, as people for example wore cloth masks over the nose and mouth to, as they imagined, guard against infection. But in Australia, the flu instigated a whole new public health structure, and so there the pandemic had important historical as well as demographic consequences.

Model Diseases:
Black Death, Tuberculosis, Syphilis

The appearance of new epidemics in the late twentieth century, particularly influenzas and HIV/AIDS, has stimulated historians' (and the public's) interest in plagues of the past. A great deal of literature has appeared on the Great Plague, later named the Black Death. This plague was the most feared disease in Western countries beginning in 1346/7. It swept across Europe, producing demographic catastrophe. Two-thirds of the population of Norway perished, and other areas suffered to a comparable extent. People continued for centuries to be acquainted with it, for visitations came more than once in many lifetimes up into the eighteenth century. After that, the plague showed up sporadically, right through the twentieth century, and historians are still reconstructing, for example, very serious outbreaks that came to South and East Asia from the 1890s to the 1920s.

At the beginning, a classic pattern appeared. News would come of the plague in distant areas, spreading well-founded fear ahead of infection. Then local people would start showing symptoms, including not only buboes but skin hemorrhages and other general signs of illness. Death would come in three days. If a person survived, sores accompanying or following the disease could turn nasty. The disease, while generally recognizable, varied in pattern and effect locally and over time. Indeed, historians have written about eras in the history of the disease and also about long-term trends in that history.

No aspect of society seemed immune from effects of the plague. How could it be otherwise when, as eyewitness

Giovanni Boccaccio wrote in *The Decameron* of events in Florence, "Many ended their lives in the public streets, during the day or at night, while many others who died in their homes were discovered dead by their neighbors only by the smell of their decomposing bodies. The city was full of corpses." The initial economic impact of the death rate was enormous: was the effect economically depressing in Western Europe, or did it cause ruinous inflation and consequent political change, or both? Religious beliefs were affected, and historians have posited endless additional cultural and social changes.

As later scientists worked out the biology of the plague, which they believed included rats and lice as intermediary vectors, even more controversy developed. A bubonic version, marked by buboes, or swollen lymph glands, was clearly described, but a pneumonic version, probably spread by droplet infection, complicated (and still complicates) the attempts of historians to construct a narrative. Indeed, the plague may have been, so one current argument goes, a series of biologically quite distinct diseases all read as one. Particularly unsettling is recent historical evidence that centuries ago the disease spread from person to person, unlike the modern rat-lice plague with which the Black Death has been equated.

Not all diseases are as colorful as "the plague." It is true that future historians may take great interest in what is arguably the most feared disease of the present, Ebola fever, which initiates a fever and then liquefies one's internal organs. But now historians are showing the most interest in tuberculosis. Tuberculosis a century ago was killing each year two people out of 1,000 in the United States and Britain, but the disease appeared to have been controlled, at least temporarily, by antibiotics, beginning in the middle of the twentieth century.

The startling resurgence and expansion in the history of tuberculosis have been fueled by news of resistant strains, important endemic occurrences in developing countries, and suggestive parallels with another debilitating, infectious chronic disease, HIV/AIDS. For millennia, tuberculosis incurred high levels of death and disability worldwide. And, above all, the social and cultural effects were profound.

Thomas Mann in 1924 published a famous novel, *The Magic Mountain*, in which he used a tuberculosis hospital as a metaphor for the sick civilization of Europe.

Tuberculosis illustrates at an extreme the ways in which many types of medical history can contribute to the history of any single disease. Tuberculosis was well known in ancient times. Since the pathogen can affect virtually all organs and tissues in the body, medical teachers for a long time held that anyone who knew tuberculosis would know all of medicine. Much the same can be said of historians who know the history of the disease. One type of history traces the discoveries (not always accepted by contemporaries) of the way in which each separate kind of tuberculosis came into the medical literature and then in the nineteenth century came to be considered part of the disease: tuberculosis of the spine, known as Pott's disease, as early as 1816; of the kidneys in 1837; of the skin in 1873. The identification of the bacillus by Robert Koch in 1882, and the ensuing controversy, make an absorbing story, along with the revelation that most of Queen Victoria's cows had bovine tuberculosis, spreading the disease through milk to many healthy children. Just the idea that tuberculosis was contagious required a huge reorientation of both medical and lay thinking in the late nineteenth century. A hereditary degeneration suddenly became an infectious inflammation. Historians are still exploring the implications of that change as well.

Tuberculosis has additionally inspired many historians because they can argue that the disease not only had profound and often devastating social effects, such as stigma and poverty, but also was produced by social factors. That is, many or all people in the growing cities were exposed. Why did poor people and women suffer more than other people? Why, and how, did the disease thrive in conditions of poverty and crowding? To what extent were contemporaries correct in blaming overwork, faulty housing, and malnutrition? In the early twentieth century, people who believed that social factors were involved in causing the disease carried medicine into social reform and new kinds of health reform.

Yet, at this same time, the mortality rate from tuberculosis (but not necessarily the incidence of the disease) was declining dramatically (and scholars have strong disagreements about why). Moreover, the organisms that were distinctive in the disease were evolving to adapt to the changing conditions of the people who hosted them. The very complexity of factors has attracted some of the best historians – and no doubt more will follow.

The somewhat parallel history of syphilis has been a mine-field of controversy. Was it endemic – and where? – before Europeans noticed it after Columbus in 1496 returned from his second voyage? Many scholars believe that "the great pox" was a return gift from Native Americans to the Europeans who brought them so many devastating diseases. But was it really what later was identified as syphilis? I shall return to this question in another context.

Mercury was used as a specific cure beginning with the contentious itinerant sixteenth-century physician Paracelsus, who, traditionally, introduced metals into the standard pharmaceutical treatments, alongside vegetable preparations. (An old warning slogan was, "One night with Venus, and a life-time with Mercury.") Was mercury actually effective? How did it happen that calomel (a mercurial substance) was used in traditional Chinese medicine to treat syphilis? Historians and scientists are still arguing among themselves about all of these questions.

We have a fairly good chronology of which physicians defined syphilis, and how and when, but the questions go on. Why did John Hunter of London, who infected himself as an experiment in 1767, develop gonorrhea as well as syphilis, so that in the nineteenth century the French physician Philip Ricord had to separate the two diseases again? Did Jean Alfred Fournier actually establish the connection of general paresis (delayed tertiary syphilis of the brain) to syphilis with clinical evidence in the 1890s? Did campaigns against prostitution succeed in curbing syphilis? Why did moral campaigns to check sexually transmitted diseases wither in the mid-twentieth century? While the questions go on and on, parallels to other infectious diseases, including especially tuberculosis and HIV/AIDS, intrude themselves. It is no wonder that, sexual transmission aside, syphilis has generated continuing historical interest.

As plague, tuberculosis, and syphilis suggest, the history of diseases can develop endless problems and rewards. Historians tend to pick favorites among diseases of the past. Perhaps it might be dislocation of the shoulder (has there been any change in incidence, conceptualization, or, indeed, treatment since the surgeon Ambroise Paré wrote in the sixteenth century?). In addition to the drama of the patients or communities affected by one malady or another, one's whole approach to medical history is influenced by the paradigmatic, model diseases on which one focuses.

Types of Diseases

The Cambridge World History of Human Disease lists 158 "major" diseases. Sometimes a historian can find a disease with a dramatic history that one can rescue from neglect. There was, for example, acrodynia, or the mysterious "pink disease" that usually occurred in children in epidemic form. Acrodynia was later reconstructed and perceived as chronic mercury poisoning, a story that has recently attracted historians. But most of the written history of diseases has consisted of extending and deepening understanding of the ways in which a well-known malady has a hidden history, or effects and implications that earlier investigators could not or did not perceive. Gout continues to inspire both social and technical history. Some historians believe the term originally covered what is now considered arthritis. Or what about phlebitis? Was it really a modern problem, brought on by sedentary lifestyles? Similarly, some excellent historians continue to investigate the conceptual and social histories of the deficiency diseases noted above in connection with ideas about the body, typically illnesses caused by lack of dietary elements or insufficient or excessive internal secretions.

Historians as well as clinicians, as I have suggested already, found that it made a difference if a disease was acute or if it was chronic. Indeed, chronic diseases came to predominate in developed countries after about 1920, but the health care systems in those countries were designed for acute disease patients, as I shall note below in sections on social institutions. As historian Gerald Grob points out, medical social workers, a new factor at the beginning of the twentieth century, were important in calling physicians' attention to the dominance and importance of chronic disease.[4] Altogether, what happened in the histories of chronic diseases is therefore a field only recently being well cultivated: most notoriously in the histories of cancers and circulatory disease (why did the mortality rate from heart disease decline in the late twentieth century?).

Other special categories of disease have also attracted historians. Diseases and injuries associated with military history have a long and honorable place in the history of medicine. For the ordinary soldier, there were not only typhus, "trench mouth" (a vicious oral infection), and other contagious diseases, but different kinds of gunshot wounds caused by new kinds of weapons. In the nineteenth century, virulent infections caused many deaths among military personnel. One horrified army physician described a case of "hospital gangrene": "A slight flesh wound began to show a gray edge of slough, and within two hours we saw this widening at the rate of half an inch an hour, and deepening." The loss of life from this variety of infection was staggering.

Occupational diseases, which were closely related to other environmental disorders, have only recently stimulated more than very specialized historical investigations. Byssinosis (brown lung disease attributed to cotton, flax, and hemp dust) was identified by a British physician in 1877, but when it actually began to claim victims is a matter of contention. Except for work on the fascinating history of surgical repairs, the history of industrial accidents – indeed, any accidents at all – is almost unexplored territory.

Some scholars, worried about ethics or technology, have begun looking at illnesses that medical treatment caused, so-called iatrogenic diseases. In the early nineteenth century, mercury in the form of calomel was administered internally to the point that it destroyed patients' teeth and jaws. Or, after World War II, in newly affluent medical systems, including the British National Health Service, physicians found that the oxygen they were administering to premature newborns, to increase the chances that they would survive, caused a new type of blindness (retrolental fibroplasia) in many of those babies.

One never knows which disease that recently has been little diagnosed will suddenly appear to some investigator to have an exciting history or a history that ties into scientific, social, intellectual, or general history. Arthritic diseases, for example, can appear to be merely a source of discomfort for older people, who in all eras frequently complained anyway. Yet the record of young people's suffering extended periods of exposure in armies in the past shows that such affections could be disabling in that population group. Paleopathologists and anthropologists can also demonstrate how varieties of arthritic afflictions attacked men and women differently, depending on what muscles and limbs they used most frequently and stressfully. And the changing image of arthritic disorders also underlines the ways in which morbidity (perceived illness) and disability came to constitute a better measure of "health" than did death rates.

Categories of Historical Interest

Some historians disdain fads or exceptions. Why study the history of diseases that are current, such as lower back pain or athletic injuries, when one could deal with serious persistent problems such as urinary tract stones, throat infections, acute malnutrition, or pneumonia? It is true that the history of virtually any disease has historical significance. Historians have in general, however, paid special attention to maladies that fall into several categories:

(1) Diseases that changed biologically – typically based on organisms and viruses that mutated over time. Tuberculosis was one obvious example, as historians are still disputing whether or not the disease became less acute and dangerous in the late nineteenth and early twentieth centuries. Syphilis apparently became especially virulent in Europe around 1500, regardless of whether the infection came from America or was already present on the Eurasian continent. And there are already a number of less familiar examples. Peter English has recently tracked the ways in which rheumatic fever changed biologically in the nineteenth and twentieth

centuries, probably one reason one today seldom hears
of rheumatic fever, which has been reconceptualized into a
distinctive streptococcal infection.[5]

(2) Diseases that appeared and disappeared from standard medical conceptualizations of Europeanized countries
(and systematic work on non-Western cultures is needed).
Historians are currently trying to figure out why leprosy
(Hansen's disease) faded from Europe after medieval times.
Or whether chickenpox was distinguished from other diseases in the sixteenth century or in the eighteenth. Or why
"erysipelas" was so slow to be identified. Was it different from
pyemia? Was it a staphylococcal infection or a streptococcal
infection? Did the organism become more and then less virulent over time? And then there was gout, which bafflingly
began to appear only in the eighteenth century in Britain.
Historians also argue about whether or not tertiary syphilis
was new in the early nineteenth century (why were no cases
reported previously?) and, similarly, whether or not diphtheria and scarlet fever existed before the eighteenth century.

Polio, about which much has been written, appeared in
developed countries only after sewage disposal had made
considerable progress. Up until that time, most infants were
exposed to the pathogen, so it is believed, and so they had
developed immunity, with the result that polio did not appear
among adult populations. Then people who were not exposed
were suddenly participating in epidemics of the disease. In
1916, New York City had 9,000 cases and more than 2,400
deaths. As a witness reported, "Mothers are so afraid that
most of them will not even let the children enter the streets,
and some will not even have a window open. In one house
the only window was stuffed with rags so that 'the disease'
could not come in."

Perhaps the most famous disease that appeared suddenly
and then vanished was the English sweat. Between 1485 and
1551, the British Isles were ravaged by an epidemic fever
accompanied by profuse sweating. In the words of one chron-
icle, "Sudainly there came a plague of sickness called the
Swetyng Sickness . . . This malady was so cruell that it
killed some within three houres." The Venetian ambassador
reported, "This disease makes very quick progress proving

fatal in 24 hours at the furthest ... The patients experience nothing but a profuse sweat, which dissolves the frame." Historians continue to explore this baffling syndrome, which disappeared as suddenly as it came. Why was it limited in time and place? And what was it? Was it a pathogen that destroyed so many of its host organisms (humans) that it could not survive?

The diseases that were redefined out of existence are also endlessly intriguing, even beyond masturbation: chlorosis (apparently a dietary deficiency in young females whose skin took on a greenish cast), for example, or the standard cause of death for centuries, "fever." Beginning in the nineteenth century, clinicians described Alzheimer's disease as senile or presenile dementia, but it did not acquire its present identity until Alois Alzheimer established an organic pathological picture – and even then the syndrome was repeatedly redefined in the century afterward (sometimes with the help of Alzheimer "patient support groups").

(3) Diseases with interesting or controversial epidemiologies. A large number of authors have tried to identify which diseases, besides possibly syphilis, came to Europe from the western hemisphere after 1492. Among historical diseases with arresting epidemiologies, the most notorious is probably cholera, the spread of which historians still trace with fascination (as is explained further as a discovery, below). Typhoid generated any number of quite real detective stories – how, for example, in the early twentieth century an epidemic in a New England town was traced to the town water reservoir, thence to an outdoor privy on a farm in the reservoir water catchment area, and thence to one single carrier in the family using that privy. Typhus, which was systematically confused with typhoid until almost the middle of the nineteenth century, was already being described as gaol (jail) fever, military fever, camp fever, and ship fever, all suggesting the crowded conditions under which (as was determined only in 1909) lice could spread it easily. And of course one of the great stories of epidemiology was the startling statistical argument of the 1950s that smoking was a causal factor in cancer of the lung. Still another kind of example is offered by sleeping sickness, for recent science is, relatively,

not well advanced in elucidating this condition, but it is still possible to write a history of the disease. It appeared in European records at least in the fourteenth century. As either an epidemic or an endemic disease it could threaten local economies and social organizations.

(4) Diseases with special or dramatic historical courses. In addition to new diseases like the Black Death and discontinued categories, there are many special stories. Smallpox, for example, requires a human host. Therefore it could spread in a terrifying way (as it did spectacularly in the seventeenth century among the Amerindian populations) but ultimately yield to medical preventive measures. Yet measles could have similar effects. And already there is a very substantial historical literature on HIV/AIDS. Similarly, allergies have begun to attract historians as the incidence has appeared to increase markedly. Diseases such as yellow fever and cholera generated special interest because they were episodic, but, even more significantly, when they came, the death rate was such that, as in the Black Death, corpses piled up and were dramatically visible.

(5) Diseases with physical manifestations that had interesting social effects – again beyond the Black Death. The deficiency diseases, once they were identified in the early twentieth century, changed the ways that people ate, and in the process convulsed the agricultural economy of at least the United States by enriching some farmers (vegetable, fruit, and dairy) and impoverishing others (wheat). Beriberi had devastating social effects in many countries, especially in China and Japan in the late nineteenth and early twentieth centuries.

In the trans-Appalachian United States in the nineteenth century, an epidemic disease affected many localities – to the extent that whole towns in such states as Indiana were deserted by the surviving inhabitants. This disease was called the milk sick, and it was prominent in the culture at the time – President Abraham Lincoln's mother had died of it. Yet it faded away. Only in the 1920s did investigators show that when cows ate a common weed, the white snakeroot, it poisoned the milk and caused an often fatal acidosis in cattle as well as humans. As agriculture expanded, the weed receded, and so the disease ended except as a curiosity. But people of the nineteenth century knew the milk sick as a major social problem.

(6) Diseases that were in themselves general categories of biological existence – like "old age." For endless generations, as intriguing historical investigations reveal, physicians explained many infants' deaths as "failure to thrive." A more elegant term, cachexia, was sometimes used in the nineteenth century to indicate a condition of general ill health. While usually associated with some cause or imagined cause, such as cancerous cachexia or jail cachexia, the term could function as a disease label for – extremely bad health. More concrete biological categories appeared in the form of constitutional physical defects. Physicians from ancient times reported "monsters," or described people born without a limb or most of the brain, or with incapacitating organ deformities, or with a harelip, or with sensory defects such as blindness. Disproportionate numbers of cases of children who had ambiguous external sexual organs appeared in medical publications. How did doctors of one time or another handle such patients? Again, a large, rich historical literature exists and is growing.

The foregoing categories do not include the conceptual history of diseases, many of which were completely transformed as medical thinkers saw them in new ways. Melancholia, a humoral imbalance, in medieval times became acedia – sinful sloth and surliness – and later changed into pathological depression. Or, a later type of example, the diarrheas, which, with pathological anatomy and other types of study, over time broke down into a multitude of categories such as Crohn's disease, irritable bowel syndrome, and amebic and bacillary dysenteries. Gastric ulcers changed from a stress disease to a late victory (1983) for germ theory. Endocrine disorders obviously were not possible as such until the idea of endocrine products came into existence.

In recent years, as I have suggested already, historians with fresh questions and perspectives have shown how diseases affecting women, or affecting men and women differently, can generate whole new histories. Afflictions as different as gendered eating disorders and breast cancer have stimulated a remarkable amount of continuing historical publication.

Historical reconceptualizations constitute only a part of the intellectual history of diseases. In the next chapter, I take up the excitement of research and discovery, including the excitement of describing or making sense of specific disease entities. Historical thinkers have in addition pointed out that the larger categories of disease changed. In the early nineteenth century, a very large class of "functional diseases" filled medical discussions, only to fade away as more specific definitions, based on pathological study, appeared. The very idea of a functional disease has occasioned any number of historical investigations into the ways in which healers applied physiological, as opposed to anatomical, thinking to a variety of diseases.

Retrospective Diagnosis

The most persistently controversial subject in the history of medicine continues to be the extent to which, using the clinical criteria of today (or any earlier "today"), one can decide what disease someone in the past was describing. Making a diagnosis of people who are long dead – retrospective diagnosis is the common term – virtually always opens up controversy. Not only historians of medicine but physicians in general and even the general public show persistent interest in such questions. Was the worm in the Bible the same as a modern worm? Plagues, even when they were relatively clearcut syndromes, have given rise to endless disagreements about what modern equivalent caused the illnesses. Was the English sweat a hantavirus?

The collaborative work of three historians on "the French disease" or "the great pox" in Renaissance Europe faces the controversy squarely. Their history of this disease, they assert, "is not a history of syphilis." Instead, they examine how groups of people tried to deal with what most perceived as a new disease. Moreover, in the course of physicians' working through a multiplicity of strategies, medicine changed, the authors maintain, and became more practical during the sixteenth century.[6] This story, using the words and outlooks of people of that time, is remarkably different from a parallel narrative that assumes that what the people around 1500 were dealing with was versions of a biological phenomenon that people today know as syphilis. Given the many different accounts from that era, who can be sure? And yet if it was syphilis, the more conventional account of the impact of a new biological phenomenon is also intriguing and explains much of the historical record.

Disagreements intensify as one takes up individual people's cases. Charles Darwin's mysterious functional illness, which periodically incapacitated him, has been authoritatively identified as almost as many afflictions as there have been historical writers; the two most prominent suggestions have been Chagas' disease, a serious treponemic infection found in South America, and psychosomatic disturbances. Herod the Great appears in surviving historical accounts to have suffered from swellings, fever, itching, pain, worms, and other symptoms. Looking back, one can ask: did he have diabetes, amebic dysentery, congestive heart failure, cancer, guinea worm – or a combination of several or all of these possible diseases?

The arguments sharpen, if possible, when one asks: of what disease did each famous person die? Accidental or deliberate poisoning has to be confirmed or eliminated for many, including Napoleon and other rulers, or even John Constable, the English painter. Then the fun begins. If one eliminates poisoning, from what bodily infirmity or attacking disease did any historical figure die at a critical time, from ancient Egyptian pharaohs to composers Mozart and Schubert?

Always the social and cultural milieu of any era affected the history of any disease. In ancient times, ideals of moderation in living suggested that diseases represented extremes. A similar guide to health based on traditional Chinese ideas of yin and yang has drawn historians into the history of Chinese thought, in which yin and yang are embedded, perhaps more than into the history of medicine. Closer to our own time, areas of recent topical interest include not only allergic reactions but other afflictions reflecting concern with the body, on one hand, and technology and the environment, on the other – the effects of air pollution, radiation, electro-magnetic fields, volcanic ash, and above all pesticides and synthetic chemicals (a subject to which I shall allude also in discussing the social aspects of medicine).

Other types of environmental factors have played into historical accounts of diseases. To what extent did settlement, drainage, and especially urbanization curb mosquito breeding so that in many areas malaria and yellow fever declined or disappeared – even before there was knowledge of insect vectors? Historians have also taken great interest in disease and death in the urban areas that sprang up and grew from the Middle Ages to the twentieth century, areas in which there were appalling conditions of impure water, lack of sewage and garbage disposal, constant exposure to travelers, crowding, and contaminated food. Each environmental condition has called forth separate histories, such as that of the pure milk movement, when unwholesome milk was killing many babies, especially when the economic need for women to work caused commercial cow's milk to be substituted for breast feeding.

Narratives of Disease

Of course it is conceivably possible also to make a disease a protagonist in the drama. Certainly enough suspense was involved. Would polio be able to flourish without killing so many of its hosts that it would become ecologically unsustainable? Could tuberculosis, or syphilis, or whooping cough heroically overcome the biological warfare humans waged against the organism? Medical historians are too aware of human suffering to construct many such dark narratives, or to try to form a staphylococcus fan club. Yet the very existence of the possibility of making a narrative from the point of view of a pathogenic agent underlines the dramatic forces in the struggle between humans and their diseases – as Sebastian G. B. Amyes has underlined in his tale of "the rise and fall of antibiotics."[7]

Disease of course raises once again the question of health. Individual health was one thing, but from communities to nations to the global village, the whole idea of damage to generalized "health" draws historians. Does one indeed use overall statistics to define the category of illness? Was death one thing, disease another? Was infant mortality – a standard modern measure of health and progress – a disease? Were hospitalization rates a sign of illness, or health, or affluence – or medicalization? Or all of the above?

The Fourth Drama

Discovering and Communicating Knowledge

Beyond the dramas of diseases, doctors, and patients struggling with each other lies a deeper drama that draws people
to medical history: the drama of thinkers trying to solve problems and to pass knowledge, old and new, on to others. Following the adventures of how people's ideas changed is not
the same as watching a car chase in a movie. In a car chase,
the immediate story ends at the end of the chase. But over
many generations, people have found that retracing the thinking of those involved in humans' encounters with illnesses has
a profoundly enduring appeal. One simply gets drawn into
the continuing story.

Ideas in Medicine

Some scholars have the impression that the history of medical
ideas and techniques is an exhausted subject. Such commentators are misled by their reaction against the long tradition
describing how great doctors had great ideas. In editing a
2002 book on *Innovations in Health and Medicine*, Jennifer
Stanton observes, "It seems rather odd that there have not
been more studies of the history of medical innovation." That
book itself is a symptom of continuing inquiry into medical
thinking.[1]

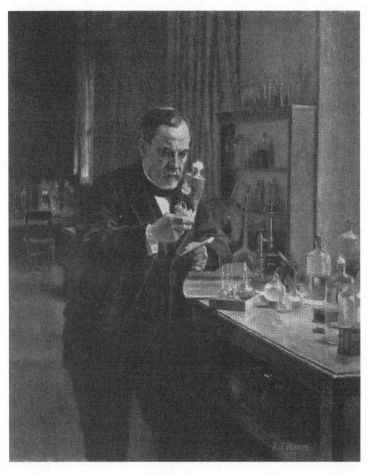

Portrait of Louis Pasteur (1822–1895), pioneer of the germ theory of disease, in his laboratory. Pasteur as discoverer and as a communicator of discovery became a legend and a symbol of transformation in medicine.

Source: Annals of Medical History, 4 (1922).

Historians have utilized three basic approaches to the history of medical knowledge that at any time identified medicine. First, historians have treated medical beliefs and techniques as one would stereotypical modern science. People were curious, people made discoveries, and people communicated what they knew. Second, scholars tried to trace the ancestry – find the roots – of ideas commonly accepted at any given time. And, third, historians have tried to get inside the minds of people of the past. Thomas E. Cone, Jr, reconstructs provocatively the viewpoint held by medically informed people at one time in the past: "In 1950, the thymus remained an enigmatic organ . . . , gamma globulin determination was still in the realm of research, organ transplantation was science fiction, the function of the lymphocyte remained a mystery, and immunodeficiency diseases were yet to be discovered."[2] Historians similarly ask, for every age: how did earlier humans see the world, and why, in that context, did they use and change medical ideas and healing practices?

Discoveries

The earliest medical history, as I noted in the introduction, was based on texts – at first ancient texts. Ultimately, the drama of medical innovators and their discoveries tended to capture the mainstream narratives. Discovery has a wide appeal. A major category in writing in general is geographical discovery – the Northwest Passage, the source of the Nile. In narratives of discovery in the history of medicine, physicians and biomedical investigators faced evidence that demanded understanding in terms of what was happening in nature. How could one explain why people in some places got cholera and those next door or in another neighborhood not? John Snow in the mid-nineteenth century believed that he had traced the disease to the water supply, in one case, famously, to a single neighborhood pump in London. Or how could one believe the germ theory of disease when one could see in the microscope not one, but many kinds of bacteria at the site of an infection? How did it happen in the Napoleonic wars that spinal injuries could affect sensory functions in some people and, in others, motor functions, and, in still others, both? Charles Bell, a Scotsman working in London, and François Magendie, of Bordeaux, in the early nineteenth century explained what was happening.

In all historical inquiries into the origin and spread of ideas, medical history shares approaches and patterns found in intellectual history and the general history of ideas, in the history of science, in the history of technology, and in cultural history. Especially do the histories of human anatomy, physiology, biochemistry, and other aspects of the body overlap with the history of science proper. In therapeutics, it can be exciting to follow the argument over whether the physical (molecular) structure of a chemical determined the effect of that chemical on bodily processes or whether the chemical properties did so – a controversy that spanned most of the nineteenth and twentieth centuries in the history of medicine.

Indeed, the history of medicine often served as a model for scholars in other fields. One of the classics in the philosophical history of science, Ludwik Fleck's account of what a scientific "fact" is, was based on the history of what people reported about syphilis.[3] And in return, medical historians have sometimes borrowed heavily from the history of science to ask basic questions such as whether knowledge advances by proving or disproving an idea, and whether accepted knowledge changes by jumps, from paradigm to paradigm, or gradually by slow, small steps.

Sometimes the drama of innovation was straightforward. We have a student's record of how, at Bologna in 1540, Andreas Vesalius, who was soon to become the effective founder of modern anatomy, in a public anatomy demonstration confronted the professor, Matthaeus Curtius, who was lecturing out of the revered, traditional text of Galen:

> When the lecture of Curtius was finished, Vesalius, who had been present and heard the refutation of his arguments, asked Curtius to accompany him to the anatomy. For he wanted to show him that his theory was quite true ... Now, he said, ... here we have our bodies. We shall see whether I have made an error ... I acknowledge that I have said, if it is permissible to say so, that here Galen is in the wrong, because he did not know the position of the vein without pair in the human body, which is the same to-day just as it was in his time.

And of course Vesalius then showed in the cadavers how Galen's description was not accurate.

Or there was drama when an investigator tried out some new therapy or technology. In the mid nineteenth century, J. Marion Sims had a patient suffering from a vesicovaginal fistula, and Sims had the idea to devise a speculum out of a pewter spoon to view the fistula. Immediately he realized that he "saw everything as no man had ever seen before," as he put it. Only then could he devise the surgery for which he also gained fame.

Sometimes the drama was more complex. In introducing a new drug in the modern period, a number of factors had to be worked out. First there was the actual chemistry. Then there was the physiology involved. One could try something in the laboratory – yet in the rat or rabbit body, the effects might be very different. And humans might not react in the same way as rats. Then one or more of a large number of varieties of clinical trial would follow (depending on the era).

At the beginning of the 1930s, Gerhard Domagk, working in a German pharmaceutical laboratory, identified a type of dye that in the laboratory had chemotherapeutic effects against streptococci. Such dyes unfortunately were toxic. One variant, Prontosil, was less toxic, but it did little against cultures of streptococci. Domagk nevertheless tried it and reported startling results in a classic understatement: "The chemotherapeutic effect which could be obtained with Prontosil in mice suffering from a streptococcal infection was greater than any other previously recorded." The details of how Domagk watched the laboratory mice, hour by hour, heighten the drama, of course, the more so because now everyone understands what followed the discovery of this first "antibiotic" sulfa drug.

The dramatic elements in the discovery of something in medicine help explain why the history of medical thinking continues to attract readers and investigators. Indeed, some stories are so good that they are always repeated, even when scholars question all of the details attributed to the discovery. In the late 1790s, Edward Jenner, a country practitioner in Gloucestershire, deduced that local milkmaids were immune to smallpox because they had contracted cowpox, which is a slight, almost unnoticeable disease in humans. He thereupon inoculated an 8-year-old boy with cowpox and found that the boy did not get smallpox when later inoculated with regular smallpox. The resulting process of "vaccination" with cowpox saved untold numbers of people from the disastrous consequences of epidemic smallpox. Historians have traced how the practice spread all over the world, but they have also raised many questions about exactly what happened both in Jenner's human experiment and in the actual biological events he saw and reported and interpreted.

Dimensions of Discovery

The drama of discovery itself has further ramifications. One was the issue of scientific priority – who first discovered something? That is, when can one show that change (innovation) actually occurred? One of the classic cases comes from the next step in the antibiotic story after the sulfas: penicillin. Alexander Fleming in 1928 may have observed some actions of penicillin, but the real discovery, some historians argue, came later, at the beginning of World War II, when Howard Florey and Ernst Chain harnessed penicillin to serve as an antibiotic in humans. Still others wish to recognize as the critical discovery of penicillin a model established by René Dubos. This argument over who really should have "credit" for a fundamental discovery in medical science will not end soon.

And, as in science, one of the ways a discoverer could gain a secular kind of immortality was to win recognition in the history of medicine. Alfred Velpeau, for example, the French surgeon, even before his death in 1861 was known for Velpeau's hernia, Velpeau's fossa, Velpeau's canal, Velpeau's deformity, and Velpeau's bandage. In the last half of the twentieth century, the often widely publicized races between laboratories to make an obvious advance, such as synthesizing an organic chemical like insulin, generated many priority disputes and made people aware of the investigators' stakes. It is not necessary to have something named after one in order to gain immortality if one's name is recorded in a history as a "discoverer."

Most medical innovations had another element that makes for a good story: they had transparently beneficial effects. Preventing death, relieving suffering, bringing about cure are parts of persistent human dreams, and many people in medicine fulfilled such dreams. One of the classic tales comes from Ambroise Paré, the sixteenth-century surgeon, who recounted how he, as a beginning practitioner, was serving in the army. All of the surgeons there used a standard treatment for gunshot wounds: cauterizing them with boiling oil of elders.

> It chanced on a time, that by reason of the multitude that were hurt, I wanted this Oyle. Now because there were some few left to be dressed, I was forced, that I might seeme to want nothing, and that I might not leave them undrest, to apply a digestive made of the yolke of an egg, oyle of Roses, and Turpentine. I could not sleep all that night, for I was troubled in minde . . . and I feared I should find them dead . . . whom I had not dressed with the scalding oyle. Therefore I rose early in the morning, I visited my patients, and beyond expectation I found such as I had dressed with a digestive onely, free from vehemencie of paine to have had a good rest, and that their wounds were not inflamed . . . When I had many times tryed this in divers others I thought this much, that neither I nor any other should ever cauterize any [person] wounded with Gun-shot.

Because, in any culture at any time, innovators usually have met criticism and resistance, these people can take on a heroic character. Everyone likes to read about the brave campaign of Ignaz Semmelweis in the mid-nineteenth century, who before the germ theory of infection insisted that physicians who did not wash adequately were spreading childbed fever from one birthing mother to another. He died tragically but was vindicated by the many women's lives his teachings saved. Many people know how finding out about yellow fever in 1900 produced heroes who gave their lives experimenting to prove that a mosquito vector was involved. And historians know other such bittersweet stories. Carrión's disease is named after Daniel Carrión, a Peruvian medical student who in 1885 inoculated himself with the pathogen. He showed that the two forms of the fever had but one pathogen, but he died from his infection. Howard T. Ricketts, after whom the rickettsial diseases are named, unraveled the mystery of Rocky Mountain spotted fever, but four years later, in 1910, he died of typhus, also a rickettsial disease, which he was investigating.

Diffusion

Still another ramification of innovation was diffusion, that is, communicating the new ideas. Indeed, ideas and techniques could take on a life of their own as they spread. What happened as first one physician and then another understood cellular pathology in the nineteenth century? How did antiseptic and aseptic techniques in surgery come into medical practice in one area or another? How did so many people of the late twentieth century find out, or not find out, about the dangers of cholesterol?

Medical ideas were often clearly defined, and the process of discovery and communication in medicine can be relatively easy to trace. Since Enlightenment times, investigators have often named publications that led to their own work, and for the second half of the twentieth century, the *Science Citation Index* permits one to find most of the authors who cited any particular report in the mainstream medical literature.

Another method of tracing how knowledge spread is to see who had students who carried ideas to others. These intellectual genealogies are endlessly suggestive. Perhaps the most famous instance is this: the student and successor of the great innovator in anatomy, mentioned above, Andreas Vesalius (1514–64), was Gabriel Fallopius (1523–62, still known for describing the fallopian tubes). He in turn was teacher to Hieronymus Fabricius (1560–1634), with whom William Harvey (1578–1657) was studying as Fabricius was describing for the first time the valves in the veins, an element essential to Harvey's argument that the blood circulates.

Elsewhere, as scholars have found, whole schools of researchers flourished. Some like-minded groups were centered in one place, like the late-nineteenth-century Cambridge school of physiology, and others were spread geographically, but each school was united by approaches, ideas, particular medical treatments, or the use of a specific technology, perhaps most transparently in radiology.

Historians can examine the writings of innovators. But scholars have much more difficulty in uncovering the readers, the audience. Students of early medicine have traced the Greek medical texts of Hippocrates and Galen through variant manuscripts. But as this corpus passed from manuscripts into printed form, the availability of printed Latin (as opposed to Greek, much less Arabic) versions generated many commentaries, and those commentaries show vividly how physicians of the Renaissance used the classics to introduce new elements into medicine. First, many more physicians and other literate people read Latin than Greek, and so medical texts became much more available to people in Europe (a Dutch commentator in 1627 asserted that only one in a thousand doctors could read Galen in Greek). Second, in their commentaries, physicians could appeal to the Galenic tradition to support innovations such as new drugs or the correct site for bleeding. Scholars still have much work to do in tracking how ancient medical texts at different times led to different kinds of medicine – even as errors in transmission occurred or as innovators attempted cautiously to appear to be carrying on tradition and not introducing deviations.

The question of audience continues with later periods. Who found out, and when, about William Withering's discovery in the late eighteenth century that foxglove, which contains digitalis, could be used to treat dropsy? Or what combination of personal contacts and publications enabled Theodor Billroth, in the 1880s, to establish among physicians that cancers of the stomach could be treated surgically?

One way of measuring audience is to ask: how did the idea change medical practice? How quickly did hospital physicians adopt a particular drug (chloral hydrate, introduced in 1869, for example) or technique or technology (like a new kind of suture)? It has been suggested that Western practice involving the use of a hypodermic needle came easily into China because practitioners and patients were used to acupuncture.

Or the same question about change in practice can be asked about a general approach to medicine. One of the richest modern inquiries concerns the place of numerical and statistical reporting of therapeutic recommendations. How many practitioners in the early nineteenth century actually changed their practice in the light of the work of Pierre Louis in Paris, who tested the effects of bleeding on patients ill with pneumonia? Or, in the mid-twentieth century – in the light of controlled clinical testing? Another rich vein is the ways in which charts and graphs first represented and then changed the way practitioners viewed not only diseases, but patients.

As "change" and "progress" took on positive connotations, healers were often very explicit about how they consciously spread new ideas, and historians of more modern periods, especially, have benefited from such memoirs. One of the classic accounts is that of a Dutch physician, Willem Kolff, who tells how he devised an artificial kidney in 1943 to try to control acute renal failure. "It is," historian Steven Peitzman observes, "an heroic, indeed almost mythic tale of inventive life-giving amidst the despair and turmoil of war." After 1945, Kolff actively lobbied his colleagues to try his machine, and many responded and developed the idea and technique, while other experts opposed it – often, Peitzman adds, with good reason, which adds other dimensions to the story.[4]

Historians of modern medicine can often document the ways in which the ethic of being part of "progress" drove diffusion of medical innovations. Pediatrician Isaac Abt, for example, described how the diphtheria antitoxin came to Chicago in the early 1890s:

> One of my colleagues, a general practitioner, wanted to talk to me at once. When I finally got him on the phone, his voice was sharp with anxiety. He told me that he had a patient with a virulent diphtheria, and he feared the child's chance of recovery was very slight, unless there might be some good in von Behring's new antitoxin. He wanted a child specialist to administer it, and asked if I could go to the house immediately . . . All that we had in this country was then imported from Koch's laboratory in Berlin, where von Behring had only recently discovered it. I knew of only one pharmacist in Chicago who might have a supply. Luckily, he had just received a small shipment, . . . but by the time I reached the patient he was very near death . . . I gave the antitoxin and we

waited ... Neither of us had ever seen its effect. The child lay still; his skin was blue, his pulse very weak; but he lived through the night. In the morning, his temperature was lower, he was breathing regularly, and color had returned to his lips ... And in the days that followed, we saw him make a quick and uneventful recovery.

This first-hand account of the spread of one of the first "miracle" treatments demonstrates how two practitioners and a pharmacist by the late nineteenth century believed that they had to learn about "the latest" laboratory and clinical "discoveries."

Tracing Roots

Beyond the models of innovation and diffusion, medical historians, as I have mentioned, employ another major approach to charting the history of ideas and techniques: tracing roots. Tracking the ideas of any age back to a series of discoveries is very exciting, and it is a necessary first step even for those sophisticated scholars who are skeptical about "discoveries." To find out how chemicals acquired a gender identification, for example, as in "male hormone" and "female hormone," one has to trace the scientific reports that led to that conceptualization. If read the right way, investigators' attempts to gender chemicals can be very amusing.

Moreover, in such a case, both the search for roots and the search for insight can uncover substantial drama, as when, early in the sequence of ideas about the hormones, the distinguished medical scientist Charles Edouard Brown-Séquard in 1889, at the age of 72, administered hormonal products (testicular extract from animals) to himself with interesting results: "The following days, and even more so afterwards, a radical change came over me ... I recovered at least all the strength I had possessed many years ago," and he was now, he reported, bounding up the stairs again, as he had not for years. While later investigators could not, unfortunately, replicate such results, both science and therapy ultimately benefited greatly from the line of study to which Brown-Séquard was contributing.

Searching the past for the roots of today's ideas about health and healing currently has positive connotations. Professional historians, however, as I shall comment again below, believe that being too oriented to the present can lead one astray in trying to understand the past. Yet much – perhaps in terms of volume, most – modern history of medicine has originated in a quest to know exactly how some medical development came about. It would be hard to exaggerate the extent to which just plain curiosity has generated interest in the history of healing and disease. How did some idea or practice come to be? How old is the use of the catheter or some other instrument? How did medical thinkers get from the catarrhal jaundice of the early nineteenth century to the viral hepatitis of the late twentieth century?

Sometimes such inquiries can have surprising payoffs. Everyone knows that when a person is injured and is suffering from shock, the standard first aid measures include keeping the patient warm. Someone once searched to find out what scientific discovery led to the practice of covering a patient with a blanket – only to find that the root was not science but medical tradition that no one had ever thought to question! (Fortunately the practice turned out to be a benign one.) In another example, with a different twist, as early as 1745, William Heberden, a British physician, made fun of some of his contemporaries' pretentious prescriptions of the traditional "theriac" and "mithridate" by showing that the ancient authorities cited by his eighteenth-century colleagues in fact used simple substances such as rue, salt, figs, and nuts – not skull moss, crabs' eyes, and the like with which later practitioners ornamented the recipes.

Looking into the past for the origins of later beliefs can start from the practice of another day. That is, researchers working on events of the nineteenth century frequently run across references to certain prescriptions. Immediately, the question arises: when and how did that particular substance (for example, ipecac, the common preparation given to make a person vomit) come to enter the standard list of medical preparations? Was it an ancient or a modern substance? Did the original use change? And the same questions are often raised about techniques, instruments, and public health tactics. What was the origin of the idea (common in the

eighteenth and nineteenth centuries) that cleaning the streets
would help prevent an epidemic from spreading?

Historians also ask how some ideas, techniques, and technologies did not gain a following in medicine. Or lost a following. Some suggestions were based on so few cases that
they eventually lost credibility. Others lost credibility as ideas
changed, like the notorious notion (popular in the early twentieth century) that mental illnesses could be traced to local
infections, such as abscessed teeth. Or the idea that consti-
pation led to a variety of illnesses. Even in his own day in the
early nineteenth century, some contemporaries made fun of
the idea of the famous French physician François Broussais
that all disease was inflammation, which, Broussais believed,
could be reduced through the application of leeches to draw
blood gradually.

The history of diseases, as suggested in the last chapter, is
based substantially on tracing evidence back in time to the
first description of the disease and then following in the
record how people understood that constellation of symptoms. But the drama can shift from the profile of the disease
to the intellectual processes of those who encountered it. One
can trace the diseases described in ancient texts, such as
epilepsy, "the falling sickness." What did later thinkers think
they were seeing? The neurophysiologists and physicians
of the late nineteenth century had their own ideas of what
was happening and what could be done to control or treat
the syndrome. Later physicians, applying new chemical
modifiers, developed new explanations – even to the present
day.

Diseases with complex clinical manifestations have particularly rich histories with many suggestive findings. Historians of cardiac disease have done especially good work in
tracking how physicians came to understand what was going
wrong in the heart. But these historians have had to deal, for
example, with apparent increases and declines in cardiac
death rates. What was happening? Was "irritable heart" a
sound diagnosis in the 1860s? The whole conundrum of functional diseases (as I have already noted, those without physical changes detectable at the time), of which cardiac disease
is exemplary, baffled physicians for a century and is still being
unraveled.

In tracing through time the ideas that good thinkers held concerning different diseases, a peculiarity of the disease concept emerges: almost all disease definitions, in all cultures, carry an attribution of cause. It is one thing to describe symptoms. It is another to develop ideas about causes. And it is ideas about causes that ranged furthest among mainstream medical thinkers. Beyond the schools of ancient times, each of the great systems of the early modern period – the iatro-chemical (interpreting all disease as chemical processes), for example, or those of William Cullen and John Brown of Edinburgh, who taught that disease was a general state based on irritability or tension in the body – has engaged major scholars for a lifetime. Of course schools or systems of medicine involved assumptions about the healthy body – as did all attributions of cause of disease.

Scholars have, therefore, written about the origins of many elements in the history of health and disease. I have already suggested that present-day beliefs raise questions about ideas of the body and of the history of conceptualizations of diseases. One of the more amusing things that recent historians of medicine have uncovered is the history of ideas about how to keep the body healthy. People in the late twentieth century (and even later!) knew that there are basic rules one should follow to maintain one's health: sleep regularly, eat well, evacuate the body appropriately, get fresh air, exercise, and avoid stress. It is not difficult to trace these ideas to the anti-tuberculosis crusades of the late nineteenth and early twentieth centuries. Further back in time, one can find them in the health rules of those who in the early nineteenth century wanted to live in harmony with nature, as they saw it. Eventually, this same set of rules for healthful living can be traced back to ancient times, when Galen and others codified them as the "non-naturals," things one did for the body that were not naturally, inherently present.

These practical injunctions for care of the body, then, did not change for more than two thousand years and are currently held holy by many well-educated people. But the rationales, in terms of ideas about physiology, varied fundamentally over the centuries, as one moved from the humors to the system to ideas about degeneracy, germ theory, and immunity. Ideas about disease, too, evolved and by the nineteenth century began to fall out into various models – parasitic, hereditary, environmental ("miasma"), poison, and, finally, the germ theory and new biochemical ideas. Debates about diseases and their causes have always been lively. One can go on, then, and ask why physicians, other healers, and the public developed attitudes and took particular actions in the face of various physical problems. Historical records continue to yield a rich, and very human, array of sequences.

Closely related to ideas about disease and the actions of doctors and patients were, of course, public health measures. Actions by governments and other groups followed on various beliefs about disease. Large numbers of historians continue to examine the mid-nineteenth-century debate about whether a number of diseases such as yellow fever were contagious or non-contagious. Since there was at that time evidence on both sides, one could never know. The consequences of either belief were substantial in terms of not only individual lives but major social disruption and official actions, such as closing a busy port.

Still another area in which one can raise questions of origin is found in the standard measures to understand and prevent diseases, particularly epidemic diseases. Where did quarantine develop? Did it work? Historians are still arguing (and so are policymakers dealing with outbreaks of animal-borne diseases, among others). Was general cleanliness really conducive to health? How did people come to be able to think that animal vectors such as mosquitoes and ticks were necessary for the spread of a particular disease?

Many students of the history of medicine have been caught up particularly in reconstructing and following the steps by which techniques and technologies, as opposed to concepts, evolved. Each surgical technique has a history. Historians of surgery at one time were the most conspicuous group among historians of medicine, and specialists in the past of surgery are still very active. The origins of reparative techniques call forth both mechanical and intellectual fascination. How should one stop bleeding after an amputation? Or as surgeons in the eighteenth century argued, from which direction should one cut into the bladder to remove a bladder stone – from the front or from below? The surgical innovations of the nineteenth and twentieth centuries go on almost indefinitely. But in each case a surgeon found a problem and tried to solve it.

Survivals of instruments from ancient Babylonian and Roman times give surgeons a strong sense of the venerable nature of their specialist calling. To this day, lancets have not changed, and other basic instruments remain the same. Series of instruments displayed in museums throughout the world suggest how much surgeons everywhere, and in all times, had and have in common.

But museum displays also suggest the ways in which technology over time became more complicated and, for the surgeon, more enabling. Right alongside the cutting and probing instruments are anesthetic instruments by means of which ether, nitrous oxide, and other anesthetics were delivered – permitting much more complex and delicate surgery. And in the twentieth century, the technology that increasingly filled the surgical theater became impressive indeed.

There were, however, narratives of many other kinds of technical innovation. Such a direct procedure as blood transfusion leads in all kinds of unexpected directions. Not only did blood types have to be established (a very complicated history in itself, centered on immunologist Karl Landsteiner's pre-World War I publications), but all of the successful and unsuccessful early attempts, which go back even before the nineteenth century, have to be sorted out.

One of the most dramatic innovations through technology was the transformation from auscultation to the stethoscope to other devices. In this case, the use of technology affected medical conceptualization in a basic way. In 1761 a physician, Giovanni Morgagni, published a book describing how the symptoms and course of a disease could be correlated with site-specific damage found in the patient's body on autopsy. At the same time, Leopold Auenbrugger introduced the idea of auscultation, in which tapping on the chest would produce sounds that indicated the presence of fluids in the chest that one could not see. Then in 1816, R. T. H. Laënnec in Paris faced a fat girl who appeared to be healthy but whom Laënnec believed might be ill, and he did not feel comfortable placing his ear on the young lady's chest to confirm his suspicions:

I recalled a well-known acoustic phenomenon: namely, if you place your ear against one end of a wooden beam the scratch of a pin at the other extremity is most distinctly audible ... Taking a sheaf of paper, I rolled it into a very tight roll, one end of which I placed over the praecordial region, whilst I put my ear to the other. I was both surprised and gratified at being able to hear the beating of the heart with much greater clearness and distinctness than I had ever done before by direct application of my ear. I at once saw that this means might become a useful method for studying, not only the beating of the heart, but likewise all movement capable of producing sound in the thoracic cavity.

Laënnec found that with this device, which rapidly evolved into the stethoscope, he could find a sign of what was going on inside the body when it was not obvious to the patient or anyone else. This was a dramatic innovation, with implications, as historians have pointed out, for a whole new approach to medicine. And, indeed, in 1850 the ophthalmoscope came in, followed by the laryngoscope in 1857, both of which could reveal other hidden processes taking place in the body. Eventually the X ray revealed even more. In each case, not only was the technology new, but ways of thinking about physiology and pathology were new – leading, in turn, to more technical innovations.

Organizing Knowledge

In the nineteenth and twentieth centuries, biomedical scientists, often linked together by common instruments and approaches, developed various styles of doing research. Paul Ehrlich in Germany, for example, at the beginning of the twentieth century sought a stain for the microscopic syphilis pathogen that would be fatal to the pathogen but not to the human host. He set about testing all the possibilities he could find. And in number 606, he found one that would cure the terrible scourge without absolutely killing the patient. That was one way of interrogating nature. Where did such laboratory approaches originate, and when?

People who are acquainted with a variety of modern approaches have similar questions about where those approaches came from. Recently historians have been looking at the steps through which controlled clinical trials were developed. Others have been looking at the laboratory notebooks of major innovators such as Louis Pasteur and Claude Bernard in the nineteenth century – and finding that the innovators' publications do not always reveal exactly what happened. And yet knowledge that reached an acceptable standard followed the work recorded in the notebooks, often with stunning therapeutic or preventive consequences.

At the present time, much of the history of medicine is being produced within the modern medical specialties. What happens, typically, is that someone runs across a diagnosis, a therapy, or some other practice that people in the past recommended. It is quite easy, as I have noted, for a person with an active mind to ask where some part of current thinking and practice came from. Who first found out how to resect, or cut a part from, the intestine so it did not tear when the incision was closed? How did surgeons solve the problem of operating on the chest without having the lung collapse? Who created heroin, and how did practitioners decide that it was useful? Most people have heard that William Harvey demonstrated the circulation of the blood, but what about all of the discoveries concerning the lymphatic system? Each of such questions can, and perhaps should, be addressed by looking at the history of one or more of the modern medical specialties.

The custom of organizing the history of medicine into accounts of each specialty began in the nineteenth century as medical teachers started subdividing the subject matter of medicine for teaching purposes. They, and others, began to think of medicine as a collection of special practices, and of course, then, each one had a history. Anatomy, medical chemistry, and surgery had long had teaching identities, and gradually the categories of ophthalmology and of diseases of other organs developed their own identities. So, too, did practices based on special groups, such as children or women or even athletes, or, as I have noted, special techniques, such as, later, anesthesiology, radiology, and microneurosurgery.

Since each specialty was based upon a body of knowledge, the history of that knowledge could be abstracted from general medical history, and so practitioners in each area had a special and distinctive quest for their own roots. Who was the first pediatrician? And who was the first specialist pediatrician in a particular culture or location? But much more fundamentally, how did the knowledge underlying each specialized practice of medicine come into being and get organized the way it was?

And then even subspecialisms could have unique histories. Through what steps, from the ancients to the present, did writers develop ideas about diseases of the lung? Diseases of adolescents? Cancers? Each set of ideas, in each specialty, presents a different challenge.

Indeed, historians today are tracing not only the history of ideas organized by current or past specialties, but the ways in which organizing knowledge in the past was different from doing so in the present and could therefore have somewhat different meanings. For a long time, syphilis was in the domain of dermatologists (chancres of course appeared on the skin). The whole area of skin diseases was transformed as other specialists began to claim syphilis as a chronic systemic infection. Or on an even more fundamental level, Andrew Cunningham has recently shown that historians who traced the history of physiology back to William Harvey in the seventeenth century misunderstood earlier writers and the ways in which colleagues at the time understood them. In earlier centuries, the search for ways in which the body was working took place largely in a framework of traditional anatomy. Physiology represented a different, more theoretical approach and was transmuted to the laboratory only in the nineteenth century, when ideas more akin to modern physiology took on that name and identity. But scholars eager to find the roots of the current specialty have insisted on reading the work of people in the early stages of scientific medicine as if they were consciously anticipating a laboratory-based and reductionist science (the idea that all physiological processes can be reduced to chemistry and physics).[5] It is no wonder that there continue to be controversies about the meaning of the work of Harvey and others.

Of course specialty history is the ultimate in approaching the past in terms of later ideas. Special competence in gastroenterology looks amazingly different from a casual observation in an ancient text that "A swelling in the hypochondrium [the abdomen below the ribs], that is hard and painful, is very bad, provided it occupy the whole hypochondrium; but if it be on either side, it is less dangerous when on the left" (Hippocrates). In the Babylonia of Hammurabi and many other historical cultures, a physician was often expected to cover not only the whole of medicine but the application of medical knowledge to domestic animals, that is, what later appeared as veterinary medicine.

Problems with "Presentist" History

Altogether, an immense amount of fascinating history has come out of asking questions about the origins of knowledge and belief and practice in medicine – and not necessarily, as I have noted, current knowledge, belief, and practice. Historians have strung findings together into absorbing narratives of ideas about anatomy/physiology, about diseases, about therapies, about prevention, about epidemiology, and about biomedical research. All of this is the history of ideas and particularly the history of innovation.

Yet medical historians often attempt to avoid presentist history, that is, history in which one starts with some current notion and moves backward into the past. Such histories can miss the various byways and dead ends that occupied thinkers in their own times. To avoid such a bias of the present, historians try to understand how people of the past used to think. In doing such history, one must assume that people long ago were just as intelligent as are people today. They faced problems, and they found ways of conceptualizing and handling those problems. They just viewed the world differently. This, then, is the approach of medical historians who attempt to "get inside the heads" of people of the past.

Presentist history can lead to distortion or even error. Hospitals (small charitable institutions) or medical education (in which apprenticeship was central) in eighteenth-century

Europe simply cannot be understood if one tries to fit either one into the extremely different models familiar from the late nineteenth century. Moreover, presentist history eliminates many of the best thinkers – those who made what would later be called "mistakes." How could good physicians and scientists and sensible observers of the mid-nineteenth century argue that epidemic diseases were not contagious? If one studied maladies as different as malaria and yellow fever, and used them as paradigms for epidemic disease, then the evidence was clear that they were not spread from person to person – and, incidentally, that quarantine was a useless strategy.

Presentism also omits some medical thinkers who were most fallible, like the distinguished physician in early nineteenth-century Brazil who noticed that the incidence of tuberculosis of the lung rose at just the time that the importation of pianos increased. He put the two facts together and concluded that there must be a causal relationship such that piano playing led to tuberculosis. Or there were later enthusiasts who thought that they had discovered the germ of baldness. Each such thinker was part of the history of medicine, and his or her thought processes can assist us in understanding other people of the past.

Historians are particularly wary of labeling any belief from the past an "error," just because it does not conform to present beliefs. Any belief from the past had a place in that past. Historians are searching for understanding, not trying to make the present look good by denigrating the past. Healers, patients, and the public of the past deserve the respect that goes to people who were trying to do their best.

Jacalyn Duffin, who is both a distinguished medical historian and a practicing physician, has written of her reaction to those who criticize physicians long ago who used very strong therapies – bleeding, purging, and dosing with large amounts of poisonous substances – writers who imply that doctors used to kill their patients with strong medicines. "Stories like this one irritate me," she writes about assertions that physicians essentially poisoned US President Zachary Taylor when they tried to cure him. "The writers presume that the patient was not seriously ill until after he sought medical drugs or bleedings and that the illness did not contribute to his demise . . . [Today] chemotherapy makes people vomit and lose their hair and reduces their immunity – and, by the way, it also shrinks tumors."[6] Physicians in both ages were trying to offer the best that was available at the time. The really interesting question is: what beliefs and circumstances led them to practice as they did?

Seeing the Past through the Eyes of the Past

There are many things to be learned from exploring the ways in which people in times past in different places would conceptualize their healing practices. Why would a really good and responsible doctor give a cathartic to someone suffering from diarrhea? What made practitioners believe that injecting a mold product into a person's bloodstream in 1941–2 would stop a life-threatening infection (even if they gave the injection a fancy name like penicillin)? Why did Elisha Perkins in the 1790s think that directing two pointed pieces of metal at the seat of an illness would cure the illness? And why did people believe him?

Just following the struggles of past problem solvers can prompt present workers to keep their minds open. When a team of investigators in the mid-twentieth century attempted to show how the Rh blood factor had to run in families in a definite, mechanical way, they were baffled because of an inexplicable error rate of about 10 percent. Eventually the investigators figured out that they were seeing, not a quirk of nature, but a substantial number of cases in which the paternity of the child was wrongly attributed!

The historian sees the drama of challenge and response as far as possible through the eyes of people who were trying to solve a problem. It is particularly exciting to look at familiar evidence and suddenly have it make sense in a new way – a way different from what we would see today. Recently, for example, Ynez Violé O'Neill was reviewing a well-known medieval picture. It appeared to depict a crude way of displaying a human's brain, reflecting the ignorance of the time. But when she put the picture together with contemporary texts and other illustrations, she suddenly understood that the picture showed how physicians of that day were deliberately peeling the external surface of the brain (as one might break an orange open) so as to establish the anatomy of that organ. Moreover, if one looked at medical texts at the time, it became clear also that diagnosis and therapy were based on the anatomy that one would establish with such an investigation. Indeed, when she had fitted all of the pieces of the puzzle together in terms of writings of the thirteenth to fifteenth centuries, she had established that medical workers of that day had a logical program of therapy based on their understanding of empirical findings, and she showed that dissection of the surface of the brain was carried out two centuries earlier than historians had previously believed.[7]

What historians such as O'Neill have found, then, is that if one leaves the present behind, and if one asks of old written records whether one understands exactly what they are saying, the answer can change what we know about the past. For the past was not only complicated but different, often very different from the present. Knowing about those differences can bring great wisdom to later investigators – and to other readers of medical history.

Not the least fascinating in trying to enter into the heads of people of the past is what happens when one replays what they wrote or depicted – and sees additional dimensions or factors that the original investigators did not see. Harry Marks has recently pointed out that great though the work was in discovering the nature of pellagra as a nutritional deficiency disease, the original investigators, although sensitive to the sufferings of children in orphanages, were not programmed to take into account factors of ethnicity, class, and gender that give statistics from the early twentieth century additional meanings.[8] Other classic works in preventive medicine or public health, especially, have lent themselves to deepened readings, particularly works out of the history of the germ theory of disease or Snow's work on cholera. There are always new ways of fitting past events together.

As good historians over many generations have shown, the history of medical ideas makes a good story and often a very rich one – whether the ideas are abstract or based in action. Cinchona bark came into use for periodic fevers in Lima,

Peru, at the beginning of the seventeenth century. The origins are obscured in myth and lost records, but missionaries to Peru carried the bark to Rome, where people also suffered greatly from malaria, as a "cure." No other medicine was needed. Some historians argue that when the great clinician Thomas Sydenham in the seventeenth century took up "Jesuit bark" as a cure, it decisively undermined the absolute authority of Galenic medicine. After the active principle, quinine, was separated from the bark in the nineteenth century, the substance served as a general stimulant as well as a treatment for "fever." The quinine narrative takes on added dimensions from past times with further chemical refinement, with marketing, with military importance as late as World War II, and with attempts to find a synthetic substitute – right into the scientific and sociopolitical history of malaria at the turn of the twenty-first century. So has a simple medical substance generated a complex, still contested history.

Uncovering Fundamentals in Medical Thinking

By taking the past on its own terms, it is possible to see much more clearly what the fundamentals of medical thinking were, fundamentals that provide perspective on current and future beliefs as well as beliefs in the past – beyond the wisdom that comes from making comparisons, as do social anthropologists. Ayurvedic medicine in South Asia, for example, has always been contested. On what grounds could one, at any point in time, argue which version was the pure or genuine version, especially later, as practitioners adapted their practices to a modernizing society?

Indeed, the history of medical thinking can lay out the many levels of generalization in medical knowledge. There were tiny little techniques or adaptations of instruments that made practice easier, such as making the mercury in a clinical thermometer stay at the highest reading. But there were grand reconceptualizations and reorientations, too. What was the impact of the localization of diseases in the nineteenth century – was the lesion itself the cause of the malady, or did localization constitute and define the disease?

And as thinking about disease went further, Codell Carter points out, physicians tended to ask, not what causes mumps, but why does this person have mumps?[9] The focus thus shifted from the disease to the human body and to immunity. Such dramas can be read in terms of the movement of ideas, of changes in outlook, or of innovation and discovery. And, one probably need not point out, the more powerful such medical thinking was in any culture, the more medicalization proceeded.

Generalization can go even further. It becomes clear, for example, that there are two basic models of accidental (as opposed to constitutional) disease, either of which may have been dominant at one time or another. One model is that the agent of disease comes from outside the body, typically an evil spirit or an environmental miasma. The other model is that illness is caused by internal imbalances or defects, as in the theory of the four humors, or inherited problems or tendencies (often interpreted in the past in gendered terms).

Only if one understands the way in which health workers and thinkers have swung back and forth between these two basic models can one fully appreciate why in the late nineteenth century opponents of the germ theory of disease often became emotional. Positing invisible outside agents that invaded the body to cause disease was simply mystical, a throwback to long-discarded patterns of thinking: invading evil spirits that had to be removed from the body by religious or magical means. In short, the most hard-headed physicians and scientists could, and often did, oppose the germ theory of disease because it had the general appearance of being unscientific.

Another basic pattern that emerges clearly from looking across many different pasts is the powerful position that the idea of cure holds in human societies. The central place of the prescription in healing practice is perhaps the best illustration of the persistent mindset that one must find a cure. The recipes of Dioscorides (first century AD) were quoted for centuries after, as with his recommendations for elder: "For water sickness, that is, dropsy, take this wort . . . administer to drink boiled, it checketh the beginnings of the disease for the dropsical. Also, in like manner, it is beneficial for inability to pass urine, and for stirring [griping] of the bowels."

Folk medicine or some authoritative source could add other recipes. For pain in the eye, "Take the netherward part of a bulrush, pound it, and wring it through a hair cloth, and add salt; then squeeze it into the eye." Into the twenty-first century, people still learned from advertisements to take some commercial preparation for headache or runny nose, or they depended upon a formal prescription from a doctor.

Healing personnel and institutions have always aimed to deal with illness after the appearance of the illness. A physician was supposed to cure a sick patient, not a well one. Yes, people could offer advice on maintaining one's personal health and even on public health measures. Yet the role of the physician, priestly or scientific, was to heal an already-existing disease, a deviant patient who needed to be set right.

Only with this insight can one fully appreciate how physicians over the ages mostly neglected public health – prevention as opposed to cure. It was just not part of their responsibility. Likewise, when some physicians officiously did give advice about prevention, they often found that their professional status did not carry them very far, for many other people were also interested in the social, economic, and cultural measures involved. Early in the People's Republic of China, government officials used public health campaigns as a response to a lack of medical practitioners – and also as a political device to unite a fragmented population.

In particular, the inefficient pattern of trying to take corrective measures only after some disability or disaster struck a society was very much part of a medical model. To this day, social critics point out that the great health efforts of modern societies are directed to often-ineffective measures taken after people become ill – lung cancer offering one model. Curing may be as inappropriate in the twenty-first century as were the seventeenth-century lists of prescriptions of substances that would cure everything from the mite to paralysis. People always hoped for a miracle cure so that the inconvenience of prevention would not be necessary.

Some of the wisdom that comes of studying what people in the past did is eternal. How should one deal with death? How should one deal with a dying person? How should one deal with someone who will likely die, given what one knows about the usual course of a disease? Aulus Cornelius Celsus, writing in the first century AD of patients in extremity, with a drawn face, cold numbness, and labored breathing, noted, "Some die on the first day, others survive two or three days." Even in the Edwin Smith Papyrus (Egypt Old Kingdom, revised in approximately 1700 BC), the physician was instructed to say of fatal injuries that he (*sic*) would not treat the patient, and to use a formula such as "One having a dislocation in the vertebra of his neck, while he is unconscious of his two legs and his two arms, and his urine dribbles. An ailment not to be treated." Did later physicians have better ways of handling such situations?

In the area of discovery and biomedical research, historians continue to find basic patterns that can help remind the most sophisticated researchers about fundamental mindsets that have assisted researchers in the past in developing useful insights. In looking at how good thinkers went about thinking, historians, again, have suggested some universals. How should one ask questions in biomedical research? When surgeon George Crile, at the turn of the twentieth century, for example, shifted his scientific focus and turned to physiology, rather than just pathological anatomy, to explain why his patients did not survive operations, he changed medicine substantially by introducing into the operating theater the monitoring of physiological processes to try to control potentially fatal shock.

Dynamic Interactions between Historic Systems

One of the most exciting areas of investigation into the history of medicine is the dynamic interaction between the healing systems of various societies at different times. At one time, Eurocentric historians had viewed medicine in colonized areas as static, unchanging folk healing. Closer investigation has shown that Western ideas and practices were interacting with local healing that was already itself changing. An ancient eastern Mediterranean prescription of the sweat from the patient's feet, mixed with excrement, originally designed to disgust and drive the demons of disease from the body, over time lost the religious context and became simply an empirical, but traditional, "cure."

The interactions between medical cultures went beyond the late twentieth-century use of acupuncture in Europe and America. When early twentieth-century French military medical personnel in southern China, for example, were competing with Chinese traditional practitioners, local patients found that over time the two systems were working together and that the practice in each one changed – often without the practitioners' admitting they were doing anything new. And in the late twentieth century, "traditional" medicine, which had formerly been a term of dismissal, often took on a positive meaning as a gentle, personal alternative to harsh, impersonal Western biomedicine.

Even in the West, orthodox physicians who encountered homeopaths and osteopaths changed their ways in order to compete. It is possible, historically, to view heterodox practices as models for orthodox practitioners – a new twist on what it meant to medicalize. And yet we also know that the unorthodox, too, were deeply affected by their orthodox competitors. Could a homeopath in the nineteenth century accept antiseptic surgery? What was the impact of insulin therapy on osteopathy in the twentieth century? Altogether, modifying ideas about the colonial relationship, between cultures, is carrying over into other types of relationships as well, those within a single society.

Historians, who focus on change anyway, find that health and healing systems have been remarkably dynamic as ideas and practice metamorphosed. And therefore the processes of medicalization and demedicalization of the societies in which illness occurred, and healers functioned, were also, so historians have discovered, dynamic in many ways.

The Fifth Drama
Medicine and Health Interacting with Society

In the field of medical history, much of scholars' excitement, indeed, fascination, derives from the dynamics of the interactions between biology and the sick person, on one side, and society on the other. Between patient and disease, a healer would, from one point of view, act for his or her society to help a sick person resume his or her social role. And in many ways, societies mobilized support systems for the ill. Moreover, illnesses and patients affected each society. Environments, disease patterns, and political, economic, and societal responses to changes in people's health status all have been in dynamic interchange throughout history.

It is, then, particularly in writing about the interrelations between medicine and all of the different facets of society in different times and places that the field of the history of medicine is expanding so rapidly at the edges – to the point that many scholars regard the interactions of medicine and society as, not the edges, but the center of medical history.

Disease, Civilization, and General History

One dimension is represented by historians who examine the idea that society actually caused disease. At least since the time of Thomas Beddoes, an English physician who turned

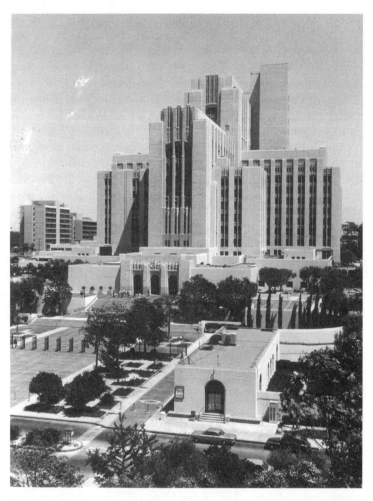

Los Angeles County Hospital, about 1979, a teaching hospital representing the pinnacle of twentieth-century health care delivery systems – and incidentally a complex, highly organized social institution important in society, the economy, and politics.

Source: A Pictorial History of the Growth and Development of the Los Angeles County–University of Southern California Medical Center [1979]. Reproduced with the kind permission of the LAC/USC Medical Center.

to the subject in the late eighteenth century, many thinkers have written of the ways in which civilization causes disease. Some medical figures wrote in general terms, romantically contrasting a pastoral past with the crowded, contentious, urbanized conditions of which they disapproved. A mid-nineteenth-century medical dictionary includes an entry on "Cachexia Londinensis," "The paleness and other evidences of impaired health presented by the inhabitants of London," although the condition, the entry continues, could be found in other large, crowded cities. Many scholars still maintain, and others contest, that density of population has always correlated with the number of illnesses recorded. Poverty as a cause of disease has long drawn medical workers into social concern. And some writers of the past were more specific in the ways in which they blamed society for human sicknesses, for example pointing out that civilization could be read as "syphilization."

Historians have also, and particularly, traced a long tradition in which thinkers of various kinds, with varying levels of exactitude, reproached civilization for illness-causing stress and various types of mental illness. "Neurasthenia" of the late nineteenth century was explicitly nervous exhaustion induced by the wear and tear of modern life. As recently as the 1980s, in Japan, *karoshi* entered the popular vocabulary to refer to those who died of stress related to overwork – without naming more specific agents of fatality such as heart attack and stroke.

Medical writers of the past amassed abundant evidence to indict their own societies. Certainly industrialization at different times and places generated not only occupational diseases and accidents but many unhealthy conditions. Later scholars could also point out that beyond poverty, consumption patterns could cause disease. On top of dietary deficiencies, which stunted and weakened whole populations, were such social habits as smoking. Earlier fashions included dying the hair with poisons, lacing ladies' corsets too tightly, or, in even earlier times, using belladonna to make the eyes more beautiful by dilating the pupils.

Ultimately, scholars conceptualized the effects of economic development in terms of environmental maladies, and, as I have suggested, illnesses growing out of garbage, sewage, air, and water pollution invariably recalled the famous Hippocratic essay on "Airs, Waters, and Places." The "Great Stink" from the befouled River Thames in 1842 was sufficient to cause the British Parliament to adjourn and flee. Beyond obvious bacterial contamination and asthma, one could mention other environmental diseases, such as Minamata disease. In the 1950s, in the fishing community of Minamata in Japan, a large number of people began to appear with bizarre symptoms: numbnesses, involuntary movements, and other signs of serious brain damage, including unconsciousness and many deaths. It turned out (in the 1960s) that a factory for years had been discharging organic mercury into the bay, and thousands of people who ate fish from the bay were poisoned. Other types of pollution did not bring special names for the diseases but created new ways to think about various kinds of industrial chemical poisonings that could come, for example, from consuming food products out of the Great Lakes in North America and rivers in Russia.

Beyond the impact that social organization and practices had on disease, medical thinking and medical care – and certainly sickness – in turn helped shape the history of societies – in ways that are conventional and in new ways that historians are discovering every day. I have already referred to the most naked of the impacts of medicine and health on society: disease events – most famously the Black Death – that clearly "changed the course of history."

There were also more immediate effects of disease on history. These consequences fall into two types: those affecting general events such as battles, and specific biographical events affecting important historical actors. Roy Porter and Dorothy Porter quote Charles Greville from the early nineteenth century: "The capture of Vandamme was the consequence of a bellyache, and the metropolitan representation depended on a headache. If the truth could be ascertained, perhaps many of the greatest events in history turned upon aches of one sort or another."[1] Of course the type of effect could be either disability or actual death – again involving one person or many.

General historians who note the social impacts of disability and death do not have to say more than that death and disability occurred. But medical historians have added greatly to the interest – and drama – by trying to discuss the particular disease process or disorder involved.

The best-known examples are those from political and military history. On one level, whole civilizations may have faded away because of disease, from the Athenians (the plague described earlier) to the Romans (besides lead poisoning, malaria has been suggested) to the Aztec, Mayan, and Incan empires of the New World. Battles lost because of sickness intrude frequently into general histories. Smallpox probably kept Canada from being conquered by the United States in 1812–15. Everyone knows that the Russian winter defeated Napoleon's troops, but it is possible to argue instead that the really critical factor was typhus, which reduced his army to a remarkable extent. The list of such instances, with attempts at retrospective diagnosis, goes on and on. And no wonder: before the twentieth century, every army suffered far more mortality and disability from disease than from battle injuries.

The whole history of exploration and colonialism is deeply marked by the impact of disease – the diseases that explorers and imperial forces acquired in a new environment, the diseases that undermined the existence of local inhabitants. And eventually the power of Western medicine became a factor in political events as well – as in first the failure, and then the success, of an isthmian canal in Central America at the turn of the twentieth century, which had to wait for "the conquest of yellow fever."

Biographical instances of the impact of diseases are many and various and offer an additional dimension: they furnish particularly good cases of what has been called counterfactual, or "What if?" history. What if a certain leader had not sickened and/or died? The instances go on and on. Did hemophilia in the heir to the Russian throne ultimately spell the end of the Romanov dynasty? What would have happened if King George III had not suffered from what was diagnosed at the time as madness – and some later historians believe was hereditary porphyria? And, most famously, the peace of the world failed when Woodrow Wilson was struck by a cerebral accident and was unable to get the United States to enter the League of Nations after World War I. Each of such individual medical cases is endlessly fascinating.

In other areas, too, such as literature and the arts and sciences, biographical changes induced by illnesses continue to attract attention. What if Lord Byron had not died of consumption (tuberculosis of the lung)? Would naturalism in literature have developed so well if one of the Goncourt brothers had not died horribly of tertiary syphilis? The whole history of jazz music is filled with contingencies occasioned by a variety of illnesses. And for medical history: George Minot, a physician of Boston, was saved from death from diabetes when insulin treatment appeared in the early 1920s – just in time to enable Minot himself subsequently to save many lives by devising and publicizing the dietary treatment of pernicious anemia.

Social Institutions

People are always aware of the possibility of illness and death – of both good people and bad. But the social aspects of medicine go much, much further than individual cases. So far we have noted healers, patients, diseases, and the development and communication of knowledge as elements in medical history. Along the way, it has become apparent that each of these elements operated within social frameworks and was in turn affected by changing social conditions.

This larger part of the social history of medicine has, on a basic level, involved specific social institutions, many of which were peculiar to medicine. Institutions have especially attracted historians because institutions make general historical processes relatively transparent and specific. Both cultural continuity and contingent accidents usually work through the concrete events of institutional change and intermediation.

The institutions of communication carried the changing body of knowledge that was at the heart of healing in all times and places. Each culture had set ways of preserving that knowledge and passing it on to new generations. Historians have traced individual instruction, chiefly in apprentice systems among a wide variety of cultures and healers. Scholars have traced also – perhaps a bit romantically – formal instruction, starting with Hippocrates' teaching under a plane tree in Cos and extending through the development of universities and freestanding medical schools down to the present.

Some great, long-lasting medical teaching establishments, like those at the universities in Bologna and Montpellier, have attracted historians who rehearse what one generation after another experienced. In the nineteenth century, the model university medical school, and one still attracting scholars, was Vienna, which for so long set the pace for modern medicine. But schools that failed, or failed for a time, such as Salerno in Italy, are also attractive. There is even a classic volume on some "extinct medical schools" in the United States – and the story only begins there.

Many institutional histories are local and limited or are largely public relations efforts, regardless of the era in which they were produced. Other institutional histories are very sophisticated in the ways in which the authors show not only the context of change in medicine but the power of social persistence, accident, and place. The history of a medical school such as Heidelberg or Peking or Glasgow or New Mexico or anywhere else, in good times and bad, contains great drama as the staff attempted to educate future physicians (and, later, often nurses and others) in what at the time was considered sound practice.

More general histories of medical education plumb how some ideas and practices penetrated or did not penetrate medical and social communities – or how some subjects dropped out of the curriculum, as did pharmacognosy (medical botany) around 1900. One promising recent field is the comparative history of medical education. Thomas Bonner, for example, has challenged the myth that medical training in different modern national cultures was unique in approach. He has shown that over the nineteenth and twentieth centuries, France, Germany, Britain, and the United States underwent surprisingly parallel deep structural changes in who learned medicine, and how.[2]

A particularly attractive field has been reconstructing the experience of medical students over the ages. At Montpellier, for example, the regulations of 1340 stipulated that a student should provide clothing for only one of his masters unless he had a credit of over 70 pounds, in which case he was allowed to provide for two. Students with over 100 pounds could furnish clothing for as many masters as they wished and could also give feasts – as long as they made clear that no bribery was intended. By the twentieth century, historians with another purpose have pointed out, the ways in which medical education centered on the student's hospital experience did not prepare ordinary doctors for general office practice or commonplace maladies they subsequently met with in their practices. And only recently have historians taken up the neglected topic of the history of postgraduate medical education: the experience in clerkships, internships, and residencies, as well as continuing medical education – all special institutional developments in Western medicine. In a more general way, Kenneth Ludmerer in a striking historical narrative has shown how laws and economic regulations came to damage the entire working structure of American medical education in the twentieth century.[3]

Beyond the actual work of instruction, and beyond the ways in which students were recruited, from medieval times into the twenty-first century, instruction that took place in medical schools was a public issue. A number of historians continue to trace the fascinating, and ongoing, delusion that all problems in health care could be fixed by adjusting what and how medical students are taught – whether in Renaissance France or mid-twentieth-century Germany or wherever one looked.

Besides the institutions of instruction, the other major institutions for spreading medical knowledge were publications. Interest in books, journals, and media has grown among general historians, and in medicine, publications and illustrations have a special place. Textbooks, medical historians have found, are special markers of the state of medical knowledge at different times. At one point around the turn of the twentieth century, for example, textbook authors included much on diagnosis but surprisingly little on treatment – which quite accurately reflected the way in which medical science had expanded without introducing many effective therapeutic interventions.

Other types of publications were aimed at practitioners, and still others were produced for the general public. Indeed, popular publications and the audiences for popular publications attract some of the most excited attention from historians. They have found many ways in which communication was not all one way, how in medicine there has always been a rich, if not always harmonious, interchange between healers and "the public," an interchange that affected medical thinking. The "public" could consist not only of the media of any period but direct patient feedback (as alluded to in the section on patients). Indeed, one fertile historical field is the impact of patients' subjective sensations of pain and the attempts of physicians to conceptualize and cope with the "pain" that their patients reported.

The technical medical publications that arose with and alongside scientific publications, mostly in the nineteenth century and after, have, however, acquired special status because they embodied and displayed what at least some groups of people thought at any time. Journals, historians have shown, were special institutions in spreading knowledge and also in developing identities for physicians and other health care workers (and this area is currently enjoying a renaissance of interest). Why did some journals prosper, and others fail, as many did? And through examining which authors writers cited in their articles, and through other types of analysis, it is possible to use old journals to trace specific ways in which different types of ideas spread. Or did not spread.

Organizing Healers

Closely allied to the history of communicating through publication was the development of formal organizations or associations of healers and health care workers. In modern times in some areas, labor unions became part of the history of medicine. After all, as technology became centered on hospitals, even high-status physicians did not own all of the instruments with which they worked and were, some scholars maintain, in this way "proletarianized."

Not the least interesting of the formal groupings of healers have been organizations that sprang up even in cultures in which voluntary associations of any kind were, quite unlike in the English-speaking countries, not the norm. Physicians were of course the most notable to organize. National, regional, local, and international histories of medical organizations have proliferated. Often the authors intended such histories to justify the continuing existence of a particular group. Since most groups met various kinds of internal and external resistance, especially from people excluded from the group, a good deal of drama can enter into the struggles of groups of physicians, nurses, and others. Histories of the Royal Colleges in Britain, of their imitators overseas, or, notoriously, of the American Medical Association can convey much information about healers, healing, and society even when the authors are partisan or provincial.

Many groups constituted but the formal face of the more general process of the professionalization that, as I noted, affected physicians especially. Healers of all kinds often organized to attempt to establish a secure and recognized place in their societies. And in the history of the groups, the specifics of that process emerge – from eighteenth-century fee bills (price lists for services to which all area practitioners were supposed to adhere) to political and social action in the twentieth century.

Moreover, as organizations in an organizational society, the groups in modern times have been central to historical controversies about the extent to which professionals could work in a bureaucratic setting and still retain professional independence. Could physicians attached to a large business or a big government agency maintain autonomy in their attempts to deliver health care or preventive programs? The problem was acute in nineteenth-century Russia and in European welfare states of the late twentieth century. Could physicians stay independent and still advise policymakers in business or government? Specific instances of researchers in pharmaceutical manufacturing establishments and of state food inspectors have been sometimes troubling.

All of the issues of professionalization continue to generate controversy among scholars. Some writers have portrayed professionals' grouping as a grab for power, or a means of exercising power against other groups, or just privileging health care workers over patients. In the early modern period or the recent period, a physician organization could play a villainous role in the hands of some historians, or a heroic one in the hands of others. But in any event, organizations mediated between healers and society more generally.

Moreover, the role of the professional was also the role of an expert in any society. The history of expertise, a thriving field, therefore overlaps substantially with the history of medicine and professionalization. Over the ages, physicians and, for example, midwives have traditionally been called upon in court cases regarding both individual and industrial poisoning, infanticide, legal competence and responsibility, and many other judicial matters. The history of this forensic medicine is a thriving enterprise on every continent.

Organizations played a special role not only in embodying the history of physicians and other health workers but also in one particular modern area, specialization. Indeed, as I have already suggested, specialization has configured not only modern medicine but much of the most vital writing of modern medical history. Medical specialty institutions turn out also to constitute excellent vehicles for exploring exactly how medical thinking and innovation interacted with society in general. Pediatricians, for example, were not only medical practitioners but instigators of many social changes designed to protect the health of children, whether poison control centers or infant and maternal health programs. Or, in the case of orthopedics, to cite an early twentieth-century example, social needs for dealing with men injured in war and industry were vital in compelling groups of physicians to take on a new specialist identity and develop formal specializations (arguably, in this case, as historian Roger Cooter points out, without important economic or political motives).[4]

For modern medical and social historians alike, the whole social project of examining how people function as specialists in society is therefore an exciting and controversial field. Did functioning as high-status specialists divert some physicians from the more general mission and identity of healer? To what extent was specialization motivated by scientific ideals rather than the monetary aspirations of physicians? How and why did the British compulsory health insurance laws of 1911 and 1948 retard specialization relative to other developed countries? The scholarship on specialization is still under way and is delightfully contentious.

Moreover, historians have been examining the intermediary social processes through which science affected medical practice and the status of physicians. It has not been enough for experts in the history of the nineteenth century to contend that the cultural prestige of science brought practitioners to embrace laboratory findings and procedures. Exactly how did the cultural milieu operate? Simply through ideas and ideals? Through management style ("administrative forms of knowledge," as suggested in a widely cited article by Steve Sturdy and Roger Cooter[5])? Could a physician be "scientific" without becoming "efficient" or operating in a rationalized, organized system of institutions? Social historians have been profoundly challenged.

Institutions to Provide Medical Care

So far I have been talking about institutions of communication and institutions for healers. There were also institutions set up for patients. And it is true that for some centuries in the modern period, some "consumers" of health services actually developed their own institutions, institutions that served for self-protection rather than philanthropy. Historians writing in the consumer age of the late twentieth century have taken special interest in such signs of consumer independence. As science fueled medicalization in the late nineteenth century, and as medical services came to look more and more desirable, groups of workers formed several types of organizations to which they paid dues in return for a guarantee of some minimum attention from a doctor. Sometimes these organizations took the form of unions, and at other times the form of fraternal groups that had social functions as well. Whatever the form, they served as mutual insurance schemes, and they could put effective pressure on physicians to lower their fees in order to win a contract to provide medical care to the particular group.

In recent years, medical historians have devoted an enormous amount of attention to the drama of how both healers and patients tried to shape and use a variety of health care institutions. Perhaps the most generally investigated has been the British National Health Service.[6] But most of the history concerns more specialized and local health care institutions, many of which had origins many hundreds of years ago.

Examining specific institutional settings brings both advantages and disadvantages. Institutional practices could hide individual experiences. At the same time, the information often is systematic and assists in generalization. How else could one obtain any idea of what operations were most common at any time? Or for what complaints poor people presented themselves at charity clinics?

The most obvious medical institution is the hospital. Current entertainment media particularly dramatize medical care in a hospital setting, especially the casualty or emergency service. But the hospital has been central to medicine, including education and research, for more than a century. Or, some scholars argue, before that. In the very modern period, the hierarchy of hospitals with assigned patient catchment areas has so dominated health care that it is curious that historians were so slow to work on these institutions and that so much remains to be done.

Hospitals started out as marginal, strictly charitable institutions to care for those who had no family (and to a lesser extent no funds). Historians have been intrigued to find many places of care in Byzantine and medieval times, or in China, where Buddhist monks set up hospitals. These early institutions, inspired by religious beliefs, underline the philanthropic element in healing and continue to exist in cultures around the world. Scholars started out trying to identify the first hospital in particular areas, whether medieval Muslim Spain or frontier Brazil. More recently, historians have in addition been tracing the ways in which, in any setting, such charitable institutions became medicalized.

In his recent history of the hospital, Guenter Risse describes the stages through which, according to historians, Western hospitals passed. Each stage continues to attract general historians, comparative historians, and local historians interested in the particulars. At first, Risse notes, the hospitals were houses of "mercy, refuge, and dying," often a few rooms or a simple dormitory adjacent to a church. In

Renaissance times, hospitals could be places for rehabilitation, and by the eighteenth century, houses of cure, when physicians, more confident of the power of medicine, became more active in hospital functioning. Indeed, well into the twentieth century, a successful practitioner often ran a "cottage hospital" for his or her own patients. Hospitals also began to become the sites of teaching and research, particularly, into the nineteenth century, sites of dissection and investigation into pathology. By the late nineteenth century, hospitals were largely devoted to surgery, while most patients would still elect to have other kinds of care at home. Then in the twentieth century, a hospital became a "house of science," and still later, a "house of high technology." Increasingly larger numbers of people expected to be born and to die in a hospital. And, meantime, it was possible for historians to narrate how the basis of administration in these institutions started out following monastic standards, shifted around the eighteenth century to a household model, and ended up with a business model.[7]

Scholars have traced not only the process of medicalization of the charitable hospital, then, but, through specific institutions, how the authority of physicians waxed and waned, and how the patient's experience of care changed. At first, hospitals were moral institutions. Later they became instruments of social order.

The social structures within a hospital, too, yield fascinating social histories. How did the role of nurses change, or that of administrators? Even the architecture of the buildings had unexpected results. In the nineteenth century, designers limited the width of a ward so as to guarantee adequate cross-ventilation, but the long, narrow configuration of course affected the basic social interactions in the institution. And on a grander scale, the hospital in each society became a symbol for the community. Imposing buildings signified public charity and concern, whether or not patients needed structures with impressive facades.

For a long time, hospitals appeared to have been the places where physicians could most easily focus on illnesses in the abstract, rather than on the particular patient and his or her illness. But recent workers have found that the story is more nuanced than a callous reference to "the pneumonia in bed

24" would suggest. Within an institution, as records carefully read can reveal, patients in fact did negotiate their status and treatment (as noted already in sections on patient agency), in the process helping to shape the institution.

Another treatment institution was the dispensary or outpatient clinic. Like the hospital, the dispensary originated in philanthropy. In Europe, after the fall of the Roman Empire, monks preserved ancient medical teachings for use on their own members. Eventually they came to practice also on neighbors who appealed to their sympathy. And slowly, with the rise of formal medical teaching, the idea of physicians giving medicines to the poor became institutionalized. Soon practitioners provided advice as well as doses, and in fact the poor were receiving full outpatient medical care. The physicians in turn used this practice, as in hospitals, to educate themselves and medical students – and, later, those taking training to become specialists.

With industrialization, large business operations developed dispensaries and hospitals for their own workers, especially those injured on the job. But eventually in the most developed countries, all outpatient services, public and private, fell into the organized system of the twentieth century dominated by networks of hospitals topped off by large teaching hospitals. Historians have devoted much effort to tracing these changes and seeking the institutional and organizational ancestors of the health maintenance organizations or various health care schemes run by governments.

In some countries, other institutions have attracted special attention. The medical laboratory and research laboratory have important histories. Indeed, scholars are debating not only the extent to which laboratory findings in the nineteenth century affected medical practice but whether or not there was even a "laboratory revolution" in medicine, as many historians contend.[8] Events and systematic approaches in later decades in such institutions as the Pasteur and Rockefeller Institutes continue to attract scholars. Personnel in such establishments and in thousands of others around the world contributed to discovering and communicating and at the same time reflected the state of medical knowledge. In addition, many historians are finding that records of research institutions with branches and stations in exotic areas like

Pacific or Caribbean islands show not only how scientific knowledge changed, but how Western medicine operated in and was modified by local social conditions in colonial areas.

Another type of organization – one of those most commonly found in the Anglo-American setting – was the private philanthropic organization devoted to patients suffering from a particular disease. The model was furnished by the anti-tuberculosis societies begun around the turn of the twentieth century. They were soon joined by those concerned with sexually transmitted diseases, cancer, and many more. Historians have found such organizations particularly interesting because the activities of those organizations cut across patient care, research, public health, and the sociopolitical environment of health. Moreover, by the late twentieth century, patient support groups concerned with those suffering from AIDS, heart disease, multiple sclerosis, Parkinson's disease, and many other illnesses often had surprising political influence.

Healing and Social Welfare

Social historians have been particularly adept in exploring the borderland, or, more often, the common ground, between healing and social welfare. Each society, they point out, had ways of looking after or dealing with people who were less fortunate. Many such people became objects of concern because they suffered illness and disability. Sometimes the questions of disease and social justice became badly confused. Why did poor people or members of some ethnic groups have more tuberculosis than others? Why did the children of the more comfortable classes, who were adequately housed and well nourished, die at least as often as those of the socially oppressed in 1890 but not in 1920?

Moreover, as many historians have shown, different people at different times had different ideas about personal charity and the common good. In the West, hospitals and free treatment by individual healers were the earliest forms of social welfare in the medical realm. By the medieval period, independent urban centers supported town doctors to treat the poor. Or, as poorhouses came into existence, such an institution would have a paid physician or apothecary. Special population groups, like the blind, disabled, and aged, also inspired people to provide charitable care.

At different points in time, this concern about care could merge into the more general public health movement. That is, caring for the unfortunate ill was added to quarantine and protective cleanliness as public responsibilities. Both governments and private groups could send physicians and nurses into centers of illness to treat poor folks who were ill. By the early twentieth century, people in wealthy communities could use the germ theory of disease to rationalize free care for unfortunates ill with tuberculosis and syphilis or gonorrhea because each person treated would be less likely to spread the disease, not only to other poor people, but to rich people.

Much of the social history of medicine has been devoted to describing attempts to bring health care to the general population in various national societies. It has even been suggested that the licensing of physicians by towns in the medieval–Renaissance era served a function equivalent to that of much later state medicine. The modern model for state medicine appeared in 1883 when German chancellor Otto von Bismarck devised a compulsory insurance scheme for industrial workers (not farmers or domestics, however). The main concern at that time, of course, was unemployment – workers who were too sick to work did not get paid, and poverty followed. Medical care was at first a minor segment of the insurance benefit, just an incidental part of a larger political and social strategy.

In the succeeding years, before World War I, health care came to appear really to make a difference in the lives and health of individuals. Medical insurance therefore became a major social issue. Politicosocial concerns were always present. One could not have a healthy nation unless the young received care, for example. But already in the early twentieth century, developed countries (except the United States) typically had various kinds of compulsory insurance to pay for medical attendance on most population groups.

Medical historians have found and continue to find any number of themes in this struggle to extend health care to all citizens. At any particular time, was medical care a privilege or a right for the citizen? Why were some groups not covered by the British National Health Insurance Act in 1911? How well was social justice served by any particular measure? Why was it that poor people, even treated free in the best of facilities, still received inferior care? And in every society, what were the particular social and political forces that shaped what care was provided, and what was not? Each theme had a separate kind of drama and controversy. Some arrangements to provide care inhibited specialization. Others, however, reinforced specialization.

The Economics of Medical Care

One of the questions that has paid off especially well for social historians of medicine has been: who paid for what? Struggles over who financed medical care were often revealing and, again, dramatic. Moreover, it turns out that "following the money" can lay bare the fundamentals of social functioning, power, and ideals. Hospitals and other institutions offer one window on what funding did. The struggle between the state and the church over financing and controlling charitable hospitals began at least as early as the seventeenth century. When, around the turn of the twentieth century, trustees of charitable institutions found that they needed paying patients to fill the hospital beds, physicians, who could send those paying patients to the hospital, gained a great deal of influence – and the medicalization of the hospital was one result. In other settings, government funding shaped what happened. In the United States, local hospitals that after World War II accepted federal funding soon found that in a new sociopolitical climate they were legally obliged to carry out racial integration.

One area of medical economics that historians have only begun to explore is the market for health care. Experts in the early modern period have had some success in applying a market model to healers competing for clientele in the sixteenth through eighteenth centuries, but simply determining supply and demand has yet to be well factored into most medical history. Some modernists have produced very exciting work on the pharmaceutical industry and the ways in which commercial forces shaped, and did not shape, health care – how research scientists, prescribing physicians, and different parts of each business firm interacted over the years.

The larger economic issues, however, remain to be well integrated into the rest of the history of medicine. After the mid-twentieth century, scholars concluded, for example, that contrary to the ordinary laws of economics, in which supply will ultimately decrease demand, in health care, if one increases the supply, the demand will grow, not decrease – as demonstrated, for example, in the British National Health Service after World War II. What part did this phenomenon, demand that could not be satiated, play in causing out-of-control growth in health care costs at the end of the twentieth century? Was overt rationing of health care inevitable? And then what happened when governments would guarantee access to health care but not furnish funding to cover everyone?

Historians of both developed and developing countries therefore are still working to describe how governments or the market or both managed, in any area or time, to allocate social resources to the health sector of society and within the health sector. After World War II, for example, Americans focused financing on hospitals, while the British, under another system, emphasized local primary care.

Medicine and Governments

In the field of history generally, political movements have traditionally taken center stage. Some scholars continue to be fascinated by power, which is exercised most dramatically by "the state." In the history of medicine, the role of governments in all periods attracts perhaps disproportionate attention. Yet one must be realistic. As historian John Pickstone has written, "Medicine is not just about knowledge and practice, healing and caring – it is about power: the powers of doctors and of patients, of institutions such as churches, charities, insurance companies, or pharmaceutical manufacturers, and especially governments."[9]

In most areas, local, regional, and/or national governments have been fundamental to the existence of established medical practice. The Code of Hammurabi and the recognition of some qualified practitioners in ancient Rome (noted in the section on professionalization) remained isolated instances. But the granting of licenses in medieval Europe set a basic pattern of licensure in which the civil (or religious) authorities granted a monopoly to members of the medical profession, as happened most dramatically in the British Medical Reform Act of 1858. Not, as has been mentioned, that the monopoly was always secure. And especially, as modernists have pointed out, the role of the state in recognizing, or not recognizing, specialist competence repeatedly agitated and divided health care personnel.

The role of governments in exercising social welfare functions that involved health care has been especially notable. Care for the mentally ill, particularly, for centuries has involved government financing and supervision. And, as historians have pointed out, if health care is a right, rather than a privilege, then the relationship of caregivers to the government is not that of professionals seeking government contracts but soon becomes increasingly that of employees to employer – as happened in some regions. At that point, medical history is indeed difficult to disentangle from political history or, indeed, from a history of general social forms such as bureaucracies.

The complexity appears in one extreme case in the post-World War II United States, when the federal government for political reasons was unable to furnish health care to anyone except special groups such as war veterans. Instead, the authorities furnished enormous sums of money for medical research, on the theory that the results would trickle down through the largely private health system and improve the national health in general. But British government health service officials shared this belief in the social role of medical research.

An area of health activity that has been traditionally governmental is that of public health. Social historians have paid special attention to this area. Occasionally they are able to show that government can be essential to health. In the 1960s, political upheaval on the African continent caused a dramatic resurgence of epidemic sleeping sickness when the governmental infrastructure set up to control the disease broke down.

The conflicts, scientific, social, and political, around public health have been explicit and dramatic at almost all times. The stakes, in terms of lives saved, could be enormous. Very often in public health there were identifiable heroes and hero ines. Who can resist the figure of the poorly paid scientific public health worker fighting against not only disease and suffering, but the forces of economic selfishness and political shortsightedness? When there have been victories for public health, the outcomes have often been unambiguous and satisfying. Polio may have flourished because of the success of sewage disposal, but historians are still attracted by the drama of inoculating most of the population against polio so that in developed countries a scary threat has gone away.

Beyond such clear narratives, some recent scholars have read the relationship of governments to health care and disease in ambivalent, if not ominous, terms. As governments took responsibility for fighting contagious diseases, officials often suppressed and denied the existence of threatening epidemics because the news would damage business. Or public health efforts such as quarantine could be used for racist purposes. An enormous amount of scholarship has gone into showing that "otherness" could apply not only to "race" and ethnicity but to physical differences that involved health status and susceptibility to disease. The sick were "others" of a kind. Were other kinds of "others" sick (a question I have already raised in connection with patients and diseases)? That type of labeling and discrimination could be both informal and governmental. Commercial medical products with standard dosages and technologies could reduce the individuality of persons and groups, and governments joined in emphasizing Western standards as in late-twentieth-century "health indicators."

Earlier in the age of imperialism, Western powers came, as someone put it, with a gun in one hand and quinine in the other. Were medical services part of systematic colonial oppression? Historians have so interpreted the actions of physicians who used Western healing to discredit local authorities. Other scholars believe that simply teaching anatomy, to demystify the human body, could defeat animistic beliefs and further the work of Christian missionaries, who presumably in turn furthered the imperialistic aims of governments. What about parallel actions to change, control, and perhaps exploit domestic groups (typically minorities) within developed countries? What happened when strong governments threatened the autonomy of health care professionals even while promoting social justice by making health care available? The opportunities for troubling controversy abound in tracing the constantly shifting relationships between political authority and medicine.

Historical Trends and Broader Areas of Analysis

Historians have in general been moving more and more frequently toward viewing healers and patients as part of a larger world that was changing. Physicians, institutions, and whole health care systems all fall under the headings especially of modernization and bureaucratization, each of which has stimulated a large historical literature, as has, more recently, globalization. And globalization, it turns out, could mean hybridization between different health care delivery systems as well as growing standardization and uniformity.

People acting as individuals or in groups in dealing with illnesses were limited, not surprisingly, to what they could do within the large sociopolitical forces operating in the times and places in which they lived. Surprisingly, for example, middle-class patients in the twentieth century could do better under bureaucratized medicine than the unfortunates whom the system was designed to protect: middle-class people were simply always better at negotiating bureaucracies. Or children of immigrants from undeveloped areas could benefit from better nutrition in a developed area by obviously growing taller, but they could also grow very much fatter, which in an advanced society made them much more susceptible to other kinds of diseases. A great deal of irony lurks in social changes that affected health and health care.

And yet some historians have been asking about the conduct of people as those people had to act within the ideas and societies of their times. How a patient, or anyone ill, responded to his or her illness raises one set of questions, often answered by following anthropological models or examining consumer movements. But scholars have also devoted a large effort to looking at ethics, that is, how healers and patients in different historical situations attempted to set standards for their own behavior.

In modern times, physicians claimed professional recognition and autonomy because they operated within a system of self-imposed ethics. Historians have been tracing the origins and transformations of this idea, which spread to nurses and hospital administrators, among others. It turns out, as I noted earlier, in connection with patient agency, that physicians at one point, typically before 1850, set standards as much or more for patients than for themselves (an aspiration that would fit into a framework in which common people deferred to any high-status citizen). A patient, for example, in these early codes was obligated, at least in the eyes of physicians, to follow a doctor's instructions.

Where more modern bioethics originated is still a matter of contention. One could always go back to the Oath of Hippocrates, of course. But historians have asked if recent standards of practitioners' judgment and behavior were a product of the 1960s questioning of professional authority, or did standards come from outsiders, particularly lawyers and activists, who intruded into medicine? Or were standards a continuation of anti-technological strains long present in the culture?

Drawing Moral Lessons from History

A number of historians have gone further in examining how healers, and especially physicians, have worked within the social structures and historical forces of their times. These historians ask a hard question of historical actors: could you not have done better than you did? Such scholars serve two functions. First, they determine what figures in the past did. Then these scholars draw moral lessons from that history.

Sometimes it is easy to pass judgment on people of the past. Even anatomists at the time did not approve of the infamous suppliers of cadavers, William Burke and William Hare, who in the 1820s hurried the process by murdering people to supply the needs of medical students. Nor did colleagues approve of the actions of Dr Charles A. Luzenberg of New Orleans when, in 1838, he was challenged to a duel by Dr J. S. McFarlane. Luzenberg, according to a report of the time that John Duffy records, was "in the habit of suspending bodies of persons who had died under his care whilst House Surgeon of the Charity Hospital, and shooting at them as marks with pistols, in order to improve his skill as a marksman in his expected contest with Dr. McFarlane."[10] And indignation continues over the medical scientists of the 1940s who conducted brutal and often fatal experiments upon living human beings in Nazi Germany or in the Japanese military Unit 731.

Beyond such obvious cases, however, imposing current political and moral points of view upon individual and group actors of the past raises much controversy in the history of medicine. It is another kind of presentism, but the present involved is a set of current social standards (that, incidentally, not everyone may share). Historians can and do argue for and against those who, generations ago, advocated eugenics. Historians can and do condemn highly compensated physicians of another time who were callous to the suffering of the poor, even medical people who acted according to conscience – that is, on idealistic grounds that still trouble various societies around the globe.

Some medical historians believe that to understand is to forgive. They work for understanding of the past. Others, as I have indicated, worry about the shortcomings of historical actors. These more judgmental writers deal with figures from the Chamberlens, who invented but did not share with other practitioners the secrets of obstetrical forceps, to Louis Pasteur, who among other things did not do preliminary testing of his rabies vaccine before having it administered to patients, to Alice Hamilton, the pioneer in industrial medicine who worked within a framework of exploitative capitalism but whose direct influence on industrialists saved the health and lives of untold numbers of workers. Critical writers' descriptions are often models of accuracy. The indignation with which they accompany the descriptions, however, does not find universal acceptance. Their effort does make the field of medical history sometimes lively in additional ways as it spills over into current ethics and political moralizing.

Where parts of the health care system were operating overtly in the profit-making arena, historians have found particularly troubling narratives. People peddling medications could be highly responsible apothecaries or dangerous quacks. Even as mere adjuncts to medical care, by the nineteenth century, pharmaceutical firms were contributing substantially to upgrading medical practice by furnishing standard substances for standard symptom complexes. At a later time, marketing by such firms could appear to have undesirable consequences, as in overselling antibiotics and promoting psychoactive substances for controlling the symptoms of mental disease in the last half of the twentieth century. Nor, it turns out, did ethical influence flow all in one direction. Biomedical scientists often brought professional ideals into commercial firms serving the health sector.

Moreover, commercialization was not a simple process. Non-Western areas such as South Asia could have their local medical systems McDonaldized (as objectors put it) by modern marketing and media. Yet, simultaneously, nationalistic pressures could privilege local practitioners, just as happened also in the American South in the early nineteenth century when some writers of that time argued that their region demanded a different, special approach to disease and medication.

Medical historians obviously have taken a variety of approaches to the social problems that worked themselves out in societies in the past. But scholars are called on to combine concern about people who were encountering some biological challenge and often great discomfort and distress, on the one side, and concerns about social institutions, social perceptions, and social justice, on the other side.

Historical material does raise ethical issues and even the issue of medicalization in general. Some scholars have been attempting to write medical history from outside the general framework of a modern, medicalized society. Some historians deny that a natural and normal physical existence, as commonly understood in different ages, was a desirable ideal. Some try to adopt the difficult strategy of describing the history of a world in which everyone is accidentally deviant, is in some sense deformed, monstrous, or ill. These scholars deny that people could be grouped by ability or disability, for each person was a human being. Classification according to a medicalized view of society, such writers assert, is therefore a biased and possibly political and oppressive act. Some histories are histories of oppression as well as of medicine.

A medical historian can, therefore, write about versions of the body and self rather than about acutely ill people. Yet healers have at times treated each patient as a human being, without regard to social role and image. Where this history may go is as yet unclear. But in the history of disabled people and the abstract idea of disability lies a clear clash between social needs and individual needs – an eternal human and social problem.

The conflict between individual demands and social needs appears acutely in the modern history of medicine. Can a society function in which everyone has to work around individual differences, no matter how extreme? How large a part of the national income should be devoted to a relatively few exceptional medical cases? How much persuasion is justified as one asks each person to cooperate with healers who will help the person leave a sick or "disabled" role? Should the blind be helped to see, and, if so, how? Such politicosocial framing may give an added dimension to the powerful historical forces that drove medicalization – and drove demedicalization as well.

Multiple Perspectives and Sensitivities

I have been suggesting how historians perceive many complex ways in which, over the ages, illness and health care interacted with society and social forms. Scholars have found at least two ways of trying to integrate the changes in societies, on one side, and ill people and healers, on the other. One is to describe general processes of medicalization and demedicalization operating in any society at any time. And the second is to see in the past the ways in which whole systems, medical and non-medical, interacted continuously and dynamically, each feeding into the other. One of the major questions in medical history continues to be: what caused the great increase in longevity – particularly obvious in the retreat of tuberculosis – in the West through the nineteenth century up to World War I? Nutrition and less crowding provide one explanation. Better medical care and knowledge provide another. Public health and other preventive measures constitute a third type of contender. Historians in this case have not fully decided how the social system and the medical system interacted.

One can focus on one part of a system or another, of course. One can come from the outside and look at health and health care from a social viewpoint. Or one can start with illness and health care delivery and the institutions that became involved. But it behooves one always to be aware of nearby historical interactions. Even specific social occurrences in the area of health had larger historical contexts. That is why it still makes sense to anchor oneself to at least an initial measurement of how medicalization was proceeding or receding with each innovation – or with change in each society in history.

Conclusion

Where Medical History is Going

My purpose in writing has been to describe what medical historians have been doing in the recent past, which we of course refer to as "the present." Yet one wants to know where scholars will be taking the field in the future, beyond the present.

The immediate answer is commonsensical: the future lies straight ahead. Where else can the future lie other than in an extension of the present? But the description of the present that I have been presenting is impressionistic. Is there any way of developing a more tangible and precise idea of the present in order to project the work of medical historians into the future?

In 2001, 2002, and 2003, the opening years of the twenty-first century, the four leading English-language general medical history journals published 205 major articles. The articles can be classified roughly by major focus:

Healers, 20
Patients, 19
Diseases, 39
Medical discoveries and ideas, 54
Social history of medicine, 73.

These journals are, of course, general journals in the field, and the profile they produce is not fully representative of historians of medicine. If one adds articles in medical specialty journals, and perhaps medical journals from other Western countries and Japan, one would have a slight preponderance of healer and disease categories. And additional articles on patients might well be found in history and historical sociology journals.

Superimposed on the main topics of the 205 articles are additional obvious themes such as gender in 24; biography in 27; and institutions in 37. Again, there are no surprises.

What such figures do not show adequately is the other dimension of medical history. The articles overwhelmingly contain material from almost all of the other categories beyond the major focus category of each one. An article on "the uncertainties of pregnancy," for example, contains material relevant to almost all of the categories I have listed. Articles on diseases or healers invariably involve at least parts of the social history of medicine, and writers on the social history of medicine draw not only on institutions and social matrices but on medical discoveries and diseases at least, if not healers and patients as well.

It is true, then, that in the 205 articles, very often medical history is segmented by specialty or by a preoccupation with problems in the doctor–patient relationship or disease in a public health context or in some other way – even the work of a single discoverer. But regardless of focus, either the writer or the reader will immediately make connections to much of the rest of medical history. An article on medical care systems that were set up by American railroads includes important material not only on accidents and surgical techniques but on health standards and on malaria and other specific diseases, with significant discussions of physician identification, professionalization, and specialization. All of this material is placed in a context of changing economics and other social changes such as the rise of large corporations. Although the author uses sources from only the United States, the reader, even if not particularly well informed, will immediately see that international and cultural comparisons grow out of the subject matter (as well as the footnotes). Or in other articles one finds that historians of colonialism in British India become drawn not only into South Asian medical systems but into the medical research and public health programs carried out there by British and eventually largely Westernized Indian professionals.

It is no wonder that Charles Rosenberg can point out that, for practitioners, medical history now serves an integrative function, combining all aspects of medicine – and showing how the elements of illness, society, and healing interconnect dynamically with one another. Moreover, historians in following any event or development break down the conceptual boundaries between pure and applied knowledge in medicine.[1]

Perhaps one can state the obvious. Disease and disability, doctors and patients, knowledge and social influences and effects are going to continue in the future. Indeed, the universality of biological disease and of healers guarantees a market for explorations of the past of health and medicine. All that historians have already written will still need to be understood and perhaps reinterpreted.

We can project into the future that one particular area of growth will continue to expand: the idea that many medical systems have equal claim to historical attention with those growing out of European ideas and institutions. Moreover, as Waltraud Ernst points out, recognizing a pluralism in medicine does not remove health care systems and ideas into a "liberal heaven," isolated from the world of power and domination.[2] Each system has a history, but the history interacted with both social change and contacts with changing medical systems elsewhere. In the late nineteenth century, for example, prominent families in Shanghai led dramatic sanitary reforms, such as sewage disposal, but while they borrowed European technical devices, they did so as Chinese operating within local Chinese social relationships, mechanisms, and understandings.

As time passes in the future, the specifics in any category or combination of categories in medicine may change. When that happens, we can predict that for medical historians, two things will follow. First, as doctors, diseases, patients, and the rest continue to evolve, there will be quantitatively more of the past of health and medicine to write about. Ancient times will not disappear, of course, but the current end of the historical development that began in ancient times will be extended. Historians have already had to deal with Legionnaire's disease and HIV/AIDS and with resurgences of tuberculosis and polio. They still have to cope with SARS and perhaps some disease that has been little attended to in medicine, such as monkeypox. Or there may be new afflictions. Or new types of patients. Or wholly new approaches to immunization. Or, almost certainly, new social interactions and institutions embodying health and healing. Already quackery on the internet has started appearing in historical accounts. Each new phenomenon will furnish more grist for the historian's mill.

When does something new become historical? Hegel once wrote that the owl of wisdom flies only at dusk, that is, when some flourishing human pattern is becoming obsolete in the cycle of inevitable change. I prefer rather to characterize modern historians as vultures, waiting to swoop down on any idea or institution that in the intractable flow of time is diminishing in vitality. I can cite the histories of health insurance that appeared only after the issue had been settled in most localities either negatively or positively. Or the hospital histories that came out in the wake of the remarkable decline of hospitals.

Yet fresh current interests also will continue to generate historical projects. Above all, anything new that comes along will set off the search for roots. Where did our new "present" come from? It took a long time for someone to look at late twentieth-century pharmacology and say that if one traces the roots of a variety of drugs, from most of the psychoactive medications to those dealing with anesthetic and allergy problems, one ends up back at the first antihistamine, which, among medical historians, is not yet fully established as a major turning point. Or surely with new information about when one type of anatomical dissection or another was carried out in medieval times, or with information about imaging and deeply interventionist procedures in the more recent past, historians will be seeking the origins of those activities and techniques.

A second source of change that we can anticipate in the future will be in the tools and conceptualizations that historians use to look at their materials. Already I have noted the technological developments in CT scans and DNA testing that are transforming all areas touched by paleopathology. And the historical materials themselves may change as new manuscripts or new archives fall into the hands of scholars.

The astonishing expansion of searchable databases is already facilitating scholarship in ways only dreamed of a few years ago.

Historians always must scramble to offer their chief product: perspective on the past. Those writing in 1950 about healers – almost always regular physicians – would have been incredulous that half a century later new histories were called for because acupuncture had become widely used in the West. Or that unorthodox healers would still be flourishing, but now with more official recognition – calling from scholars at the end of the twentieth century much more intensive and extensive historical investigation into a wide variety of popular and even superstitious practitioners, from ancient times right down to those who were equally "unscientific" but deferred to by officials and the media at the turn of the twenty-first century.

It may be, as Michael Neve suggests, that, over time, the history of medicine shifts back and forth between a progressive account of "a series of historical icons" and a search for "historical context."[3] It may be that historians will praise or deplore the ways in which the biomedical model, in which diseases were an intrusion to be corrected, replaced the earlier Western view in which disease was an integral part of the self and the world of God and nature. Even when formal medical care was marginal in society, the issues involved were so important that the history was dramatic.

Historians who consciously strive for perspective amidst the dramas run across recurring questions that continue to serve historical inquiry well. Rosemary Stevens, for example, characterizes medicine in the twentieth century in terms of great underlying tendencies, first to centralize medicine (as in setting new standards – often through examinations – for all practitioners) and then to decentralize it (as the importance of specialization and specialists grew, fragmenting the profession and practice).[4] Using such a perspective transforms and gives added meaning to more specific narratives of change in medical practice and health care systems over many decades. Moreover, those writing about medieval and Renaissance medicine may find that this formulation of events in the twentieth century suggests ways of configuring the twelfth to the sixteenth centuries, when uniting and fragmenting were already part of the standard story. And there will, no doubt, be other overarching perspectives that will inspire historians of medicine.

Historians will likely continue to have readers. Indeed, as I have suggested, "the market for the product" is remarkably promising. As long as there are illnesses and healers, medical history will continue to provide context for the efforts of humans to deal with their ailments. Practitioners of medicine will find reassurance in the timelessness of the healing enter prise and may also use history to soften the arrogance of any generation caught up in the excitement of knowledge and treatment. Sufferers from biological invaders and from environmental toxins may also gain from finding out what scholars can tell about how people in the past coped with sickness and fatality.

As social authorities attempt to solve problems of health, they often turn to history and historians. Any public official who attempts to institute – or not institute – a quarantine would be foolish not to attend to the historical record from ancient times to the twentieth century. Or one can gain knowledge about organizing and administering health care, or specific issues like the control of dangerous substances or trying to change public health standards. Even in history, today or in the future, such questions are controversial. As historian Virginia Berridge asks pointedly, "How does an 'historical fact' become a 'policy truth'?"[5]

What is most uncertain, of course, is exactly in which directions the ingenuity of historians will take them as they read and interpret records from the past (including the recent past). Many historians still write and probably will in the future write about great doctors and great discoveries. Reconstructing the experiences through which people went to devise an innovation still exerts a very powerful attraction for both writers and readers. Many historians will continue to act in a traditional role, as story-tellers for their cultures, especially the medical cultures in which workers need heroic figures and historic roots in order to be inspired. And still other historians will be searching for what is intellectually trendy at any time – so that they can have a new and stimulating way to read material from the past.

For the immediate future, it is safe to say that explicit tension will continue between those who feel the need to tell a simple, clear narrative story and those who see wisdom that can come from complex, ironic, nuanced, and even ragged accounts of what appear at first glance to be clear events. Yet in reaction against the extremes of theory and nihilism of some historians in the late twentieth century, scholars in at least the first years of the twenty-first century were moving into a remarkably tolerant eclecticism, in which historians of all approaches and interpretations are welcome. With Mark Jackson, historians recognize how individual are works of scholarship: "This does not imply that one form of history is necessarily better than another, but merely that they offer different perspectives on the past."[6]

Within that eclecticism, emphases are discernible. Sophisticated examinations of knowledge production, communication, and audience are very much in order. Healers of all kinds now belong within the active purview of historians. Healers interacted not only between societies, but between cultures, cultures that existed inside of their own societies or outside. Disease and illness now tend to revolve around how people conceived of bodies – their own and other people's, including issues of gender, self, identity, genetics, and individuality. Twentieth-century specialists will continue to look at both Western and non-Western medical systems alternative to the scientistic biomedicine coming out of parts of North America.

Institutions, ideas, and biography may become more incidental. Or more important. But one thing seems certain: medical history will thrive. And the past universality of the healing role and the medical ceremony will continue to be a striking fact. People will continue to understand that in human affairs, the confrontation with nature that medical history encompasses was different from other human challenges. Yes, mixed in with economic and social and work changes, complicated by religions and by movements of secularization and perhaps modernization. In the process, medicalization has taken and will take on a meaning and a momentum all its own.

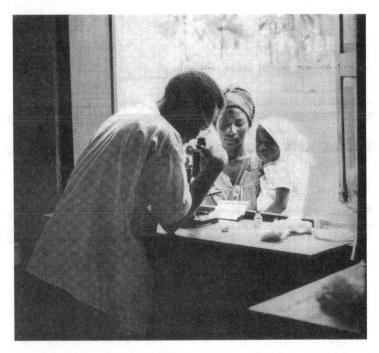

A mother bringing her child for a routine check to a medical center set up in the Congo by the World Health Organization in the 1960s. Despite any cultural differences, professional medical personnel staffed the center, which included the basic technology of Western medicine at that time.

Source: The Second Ten Years of the World Health Organization, 1958–1967 (1968). Reproduced with the kind permission of the World Health Organization.

Suggestions for Further Reading

Someone wishing to find out more about medical history or follow up some question is fortunate, for much of the field is covered in a two-volume collection edited by W. F. Bynum and Roy Porter: *Companion Encyclopedia of the History of Medicine* (London: Routledge, 1993). The contributors to the *Companion* deal with both content, such as different types of diseases and therapies, and approaches that authors take to major topics and to the subject in general. There is also now a brief and very broad global history of medicine and health: Sheldon Watts, *Disease and Medicine in World History* (New York: Routledge, 2003).

For specific topics in medical history, the field is served by two excellent indexes that do not entirely overlap. Both, however, are devoted to historical publications. One is the *Bibliography of the History of Medicine*, issued in cumulated volumes by the US National Library of Medicine from 1964 to 1993, after which it was largely incorporated into, and continued by, the National Library of Medicine online services. The other great modern running bibliography of medical history is the Wellcome Institute for the History of Medicine's *Current Work in the History of Medicine*, begun in 1954 and now largely incorporated and continued in the Wellcome Library online catalogue. For history of medicine in particular countries, usually one kind of bibliography or another exists. Australia, for example, has Bryan Gandevia,

Alison Holster, and Sheila Simpson, *An Annotated Bibliography of the History of Medicine and Health in Australia* (Sydney: Royal Australasian College of Physicians, 1984). *Bibliography of the History of Medicine of the United States and Canada, 1939–1960*, ed. Genevieve Miller (Baltimore: Johns Hopkins Press, 1964), covers publications from the period before the National Library of Medicine *Bibliography of the History of Medicine* begins.

A formidable number of general histories of medicine exist and continue to appear. Some are lavishly illustrated and are meant to appeal to a general public – but nonetheless incorporate excellent scholarship. Such would be *The Cambridge Illustrated History of Medicine*, ed. Roy Porter (Cambridge: Cambridge University Press, 1996). Another is *Western Medicine: An Illustrated History*, ed. Irvine Loudon (Oxford: Oxford University Press, 1997). Of the old-fashioned but useful compilations of names, discoveries, and basic facts, perhaps the best is the English version of Arturo Castiglioni, *A History of Medicine*, trans. and ed. E. B. Krumbhaar (2nd edn, New York: Alfred A. Knopf, 1958), which can be used as an encyclopedia. A more recent and compact introduction is Lois Magner, *A History of Medicine* (New York: Marcel Dekker, 1992). Two rich modern narratives are Roy Porter, *The Greatest Benefit to Mankind: A Medical History of Humanity* (New York: W. W. Norton, 1997), and Lawrence I. Conrad et al., *The Western Medical Tradition, 800 BC to AD 1800* (Cambridge: Cambridge University Press, 1995). And some people still like the narrative in Erwin H. Ackerknecht, *A Short History of Medicine* (2nd edn, New York: Ronald Press, 1969).

Two general histories introducing the field, however, stand out. One is Robert P. Hudson, *Disease and Its Control: The Shaping of Modern Thought* (Westport CT: Greenwood Press, 1983), a beautifully written introduction to basic topics by a senior historian of medicine. The other is a lively, understandable, and authoritative teaching text, by Jacalyn Duffin, *History of Medicine: A Scandalously Short Introduction* (Toronto: University of Toronto Press, 1999). Duffin provides good narrative and also instructions on "Sleuthing and Science: How to Research a Question in Medical History," together with not only an extensive bibliography but a list of online resources. Indeed, her coverage of where a reader might turn next is so incisive that I do not attempt to repeat most of the material here. Another brief, practical introduction is Robert J. T. Joy and Dale C. Smith, "On Writing Medical History," *Annals of Diagnostic Pathology*, 1 (1997), 130–7.

Problems and perspectives in the history of medicine are also well represented. Those which are most basic and helpful include Lester King, *Medical Thinking: A Historical Preface* (Princeton NJ: Princeton University Press, 1982); Charles E. Rosenberg, *Explaining Epidemics and Other Studies in the History of Medicine* (Cambridge: Cambridge University Press, 1992); and *Problems and Methods in the History of Medicine*, eds Roy Porter and Andrew Wear (London: Croom Helm, 1987). A particularly fresh entry is K. Codell Carter, *The Rise of Causal Concepts of Disease: Case Histories* (Aldershot: Ashgate, 2003).

A large number of books deal with healers. Individual healers have biographies, and for the more famous figures such as Harvey or Pasteur, usually a number of writers have produced "lives." Any number of general books exist, such as Sherwin Nuland's *Doctors: The Biography of Medicine* (New York: Alfred A. Knopf, 1988). Or physicians have been grouped by country or by medical specialty. An especially good series, published by the Clarendon Press, is Irvine Loudon, *Medical Care and the General Practitioner, 1750–1850*; Anne Digby, *The Evolution of British General Practice 1850–1948*; and *General Practice under the National Health Service, 1948–1997*, eds Irvine Loudon, John Horder, and Charles Webster.

Most recent works concerning medical practice also include much material on patients, as is explicit in Edward Shorter, *Doctors and Their Patients: A Social History* (New Brunswick NJ: Transaction, 1991). Other, more focused books are Roy Porter and Dorothy Porter, *In Sickness and in Health: The British Experience 1650–1850* (London: Fourth Estate, 1988); Anne Digby, *Making a Medical Living: Doctors and Patients in the English Market for Medicine, 1720–1911* (Cambridge: Cambridge University Press, 1994); M. R. McVaugh, *Medicine Before the Plague: Practitioners and Their Patients in the Crown of Aragon, 1285–1345*

(Cambridge: Cambridge University Press, 1993); Matthew Ramsey, *Professional and Popular Medicine in France, 1770–1830: The Social World of Medical Practice* (New York: Cambridge University Press, 1988); and Martin S. Pernick, *A Calculus of Suffering: Pain, Professionalism, and Anesthesia in Nineteenth-Century America* (New York: Columbia University Press, 1985), to name just a few representative examples.

Medical history now has many excellent histories of a wide variety of diseases. The key to this literature is *The Cambridge World History of Human Disease*, ed. Kenneth F. Kiple (Cambridge: Cambridge University Press, 1993), a work that is both comprehensive and deep. A very rich narrative account is Gerald N. Grob, *The Deadly Truth: A History of Disease in America* (Cambridge MA: Harvard University Press, 2002). The history of epidemic diseases and their impact is particularly well served, from the classic William H. McNeill, *Plagues and Peoples* (Garden City NY: Anchor Books, 1976), to Sheldon Watts, *Epidemics and History: Disease, Power, and Imperialism* (New Haven CT: Yale University Press, 1997).

Someone looking for reading on special topics or problems can find any number of good books covering different eras in the history of medicine. Some of the newer ones include Nancy G. Siraisi, *Medieval & Early Renaissance Medicine: An Introduction to Knowledge and Practice* (Chicago: University of Chicago Press, 1990); Roger French, *Medicine Before Science: The Rational and Learned Doctor from the Middle Ages to the Enlightenment* (Cambridge: Cambridge University Press, 2003); W. F. Bynum, *Science and the Practice of Medicine in the Nineteenth Century* (Cambridge: Cambridge University Press, 1994); and *Medicine in the Twentieth Century*, eds Roger Cooter and John Pickstone (Amsterdam: Harwood Academic, 2000). The authors in *Ancient Medicine in Its Socio-Cultural Context*, eds Ph. J. van der Eijk, H. F. J. Horstmanshoff, and P. H. Schrijvers (Amsterdam: Rodopi, 1995), cover ancient times suggestively.

Additional references in the books listed above or, even better, library catalogues provide an astonishing array of riches. Beyond biographies, there are histories of every specialization, from plastic surgery to dermatology to sports medicine and podiatry, dentistry, and nursing. Alternative practices and folk medicine also have their historians. And local histories are legion, whether of epidemics, social and cultural contexts, medical economics, or people and institutions. Sweeping histories, too, exist, such as Guenter Risse, *Mending Bodies, Saving Souls: A History of Hospitals* (New York: Oxford University Press, 1999), and James C. Riley, *Rising Life Expectancy: A Global History* (Cambridge: Cambridge University Press, 2001). A point of departure for many historians has been *Medicine and Society: Historical Essays*, ed. Andrew Wear (Cambridge: Cambridge University Press, 1992). The richness of learned medicine from around the globe is suggested in *Knowledge and the Scholarly Medical Traditions*, ed. Don Bates (Cambridge: Cambridge University Press, 1995), and *Medicine Across Cultures: History and Practice of Medicine in Non-Western Cultures*, ed. Helaine Selin (Dordrecht: Kluwer Academic, 2003). For advanced students, *Locating Medical History: The Stories and Their Meanings*, eds Frank Huisman and John Harley Warner (Baltimore: Johns Hopkins University Press, 2004), contains extensive historiographical and interpretive arguments and underlines the broad eclecticism now dominating the history of medicine.

The field is also served by some great popular classics that still often function to introduce people to medical history. One is Hans Zinsser, *Rats, Lice and History* (Boston: Little, Brown, 1935). Paul de Kruif wrote a series of riveting accounts of major medical discoveries, particularly *Microbe Hunters* (New York: Blue Ribbon Books, 1926) and *Men Against Death* (New York: Harcourt, Brace, 1932). Finally, a novel, by Sinclair Lewis, *Arrowsmith* (New York: Harcourt, Brace, 1925), should be mentioned. It was written with the silent advice of a distinguished medical scientist and is part of the common communication base in the field.

There also exists a list of classic texts and key technical publications in medicine through the ages: *Morton's Medical Bibliography: An Annotated Check-List of Texts Illustrating the History of Medicine (Garrison and Morton)*, ed. Jeremy M. Norman (5th edn, Aldershot: Scolar Press, 1991).

The major medical history journals are particularly valuable, for they carry not only a wide variety of interesting articles but book lists and reviews that guide one to current publications. English-language journals include *Medical History*; *Bulletin of the History of Medicine*; *Journal of the History of Medicine and Allied Sciences*; *Social History of Medicine*; *Canadian Bulletin of the History of Medicine*; *Health and History*; and *Journal of Medical Biography*. Some Continental journals also carry occasional articles in English, including the Swiss journal *Gesnerus* and the international journal *Vesalius*.

But most fun of all is to look at the old books and journals that provide the main records from which medical history can be written. Or one can go into archives and museum collections. But all of such original materials from the past of medicine and health should be used with care. One can be drawn in to looking at them, become fascinated, and lose track of time.

Notes

Introduction: Where Medical History Came From

1   Christopher Lawrence, "The Meaning of Histories," *Bulletin of the History of Medicine*, 66 (1992), 638–45.
2   Joan Lane, *A Social History of Medicine: Health, Healing and Disease in England, 1750–1950* (London: Routledge, 2001), p. vii.
3   Robert A. Nye, "The Evolution of the Concept of Medicalization in the Late Twentieth Century," *Journal of the History of the Behavioral Sciences*, 39 (2003), 115–29.
4   Janet Golden, " 'An Argument That Goes Back to the Womb': The Demedicalization of Fetal Alcohol Syndrome, 1973–1992," *Journal of Social History*, 33 (1999), 270–1.

The First Drama: The Healer

1   Raymond Prince, "Indigenous Yoruba Psychiatry," in *Magic, Faith, and Healing: Studies in Primitive Psychiatry Today*, ed. Ari Kiev (New York: Free Press of Glencoe, 1964), pp. 94–5.
2   Owsei Temkin, *The Double Face of Janus and Other Essays in the History of Medicine* (Baltimore: Johns Hopkins University Press, 1977), pp. 41–3.
3   Heinrich von Staden, unpublished public lecture materials.
4   Vern L. Bullough, *The Development of Medicine as a Profession: The Contribution of the Medieval University to Modern Medicine* (Basel: S. Karger, 1966).

5   Based on Ernest Greenwood, "Attributes of a Profession," *Social Work*, 2 (1957), 45–55; John C. Burnham, *How the Idea of Profession Changed the Writing of Medical History* (London: Wellcome Institute for the History of Medicine, 1998), pp. 78–80.
6   Robert Jütte, "Introduction," in *Historical Aspects of Unconventional Medicine: Approaches, Concepts, Case Studies*, eds Robert Jütte, Motzi Eklöf, and Marie C. Nelson (Sheffield: European Association for the History of Medicine and Health Publications, 2001), p. 4.
7   P. Laín Entralgo, *Doctor and Patient*, trans. Frances Partridge (New York: McGraw-Hill, 1969).
8   Michael MacDonald, *Mystical Bedlam: Madness, Anxiety, and Healing in Seventeenth-Century England* (Cambridge: Cambridge University Press, 1981).
9   Laurel Ulrich, *A Midwife's Tale: The Life of Martha Ballard, Based on Her Diary, 1785–1812* (New York: Alfred A. Knopf, 1990).
10 Richard H. Shryock, "Public Relations of the Medical Profession in Great Britain and the United States: 1600–1870," *Annals of Medical History*, n.s. 2 (1930), 308–39.

The Second Drama: The Sick Person

1   Anne Digby, "The Patient's View," in *Western Medicine: An Illustrated History*, ed. Irvine Loudon (Oxford: Oxford University Press, 1997), p. 291.
2   Talcott Parsons, *The Social System* (Glencoe IL: Free Press, 1951), especially ch. X.
3   Lester S. King, *Medical Thinking: A Historical Preface* (Princeton NJ: Princeton University Press, 1982), p. 133.
4   Linda F. Hogle, *Recovering the Nation's Body: Cultural Memory, Medicine, and the Politics of Redemption* (New Brunswick NJ: Rutgers University Press, 1999), p. 3.
5   Emily Martin, *Flexible Bodies: Tracking Immunity in American Culture – From the Days of Polio to the Age of AIDS* (Boston: Beacon Press, 1994), p. 236.
6   Martin Dinges, "Men's Bodies 'Explained' on a Daily Basis in Letters from Patients to Samuel Hahnemann (1830–1835)," in *Patients in the History of Homeopathy*, ed. Martin Dinges (Sheffield: European Association for the History of Medicine and Health Publications, 2002), pp. 85–118.
7   Mary Lindemann, *Health and Healing in Eighteenth-Century Germany* (Baltimore: Johns Hopkins University Press, 1996).

8   Laurence Brockliss and Colin Jones, *The Medical World of Early Modern France* (Oxford: Clarendon Press, 1997), pp. 293–5.

The Third Drama: Diseases

1   Charles E. Rosenberg, "Framing Disease: Illness, Society, and History," in *Framing Disease: Studies in Cultural History*, eds Charles E. Rosenberg and Janet Golden (New Brunswick NJ: Rutgers University Press, 1992), pp. xiii–xxvi.
2   Robert P. Hudson, *Disease and Its Control: The Shaping of Modern Thought* (Westport CT: Greenwood Press, 1983), p. 164.
3   William H. McNeill, *Plagues and Peoples* (Garden City NY: Anchor Books, 1976), p. 133.
4   Gerald N. Grob, *The Deadly Truth: A History of Disease in America* (Cambridge MA: Harvard University Press, 2002), pp. 228–9.
5   Peter C. English, *Rheumatic Fever in America and Britain: A Biological, Epidemiological, and Medical History* (New Brunswick NJ: Rutgers University Press, 1999).
6   Jon Arrizabalaga, John Henderson, and Roger French, *The Great Pox: The French Disease in Renaissance Europe* (New Haven CT: Yale University Press, 1997).
7   Sebastian G. B. Amyes, *Magic Bullets, Lost Horizons: The Rise and Fall of Antibiotics* (London: Taylor & Francis, 2001).

The Fourth Drama:
Discovering and Communicating Knowledge

1   Jennifer Stanton, "Introduction: On Theory and Practice," in *Innovations in Health and Medicine: Diffusion and Resistance in the Twentieth Century*, ed. Jennifer Stanton (London: Routledge, 2002), p. 1.
2   Thomas E. Cone, Jr, *History of American Pediatrics* (Boston: Little, Brown, 1979), p. 232.
3   Ludwik Fleck, *Genesis and Development of a Scientific Fact*, eds Thaddeus J. Trenn and Robert K. Merton, trans. Fred Bradley and Thaddeus J. Trenn (Chicago: University of Chicago Press, 1979).
4   Steven J. Peitzman, "Origins and Early Reception of Clinical Dialysis," *American Journal of Nephrology*, 17 (1997), 299–304.

5   Andrew Cunningham, "The Pen and the Sword: Recovering the Disciplinary Identity of Physiology and Anatomy before 1800. I: Old Physiology – the Pen," *Studies in History and Philosophy of Biological and Biomedical Sciences*, 33 (2002), 631–65.

6   Jacalyn Duffin, *History of Medicine: A Scandalously Short Introduction* (Toronto: University of Toronto Press, 1999), p. 90.

7   Y. V. O'Neill, "Meningeal Localization: A New Key to Some Medical Texts, Diagnoses and Practices of the Middle Ages," *Mediaevistik*, 6 (1993), 211–31.

8   Harry M. Marks, "Epidemiologists Explain Pellagra: Gender, Race, and Political Economy in the Work of Edgar Sydenstricker," *Journal of the History of Medicine and Allied Sciences*, 58 (2003), 34–55.

9   K. Codell Carter, *The Rise of Causal Concepts of Disease: Case Histories* (Aldershot: Ashgate, 2003).

The Fifth Drama:
Medicine and Health Interacting with Society

1   Roy Porter and Dorothy Porter, *In Sickness and in Health: The British Experience 1650–1850* (London: Fourth Estate, 1988), p. 275.

2   Thomas Neville Bonner, *Medical Education in Britain, France, Germany, and the United States, 1750–1945* (New York: Oxford University Press, 1995).

3   Kenneth M. Ludmerer, *Time to Heal: American Medical Education from the Turn of the Century to the Era of Managed Care* (Oxford: Oxford University Press, 1999).

4   Roger Cooter, *Surgery and Society in Peace and War: Orthopaedics and the Organization of Modern Medicine, 1880–1948* (Houndmills: Macmillan, 1993).

5   Steve Sturdy and Roger Cooter, "Science, Scientific Management, and the Transformation of Medicine in Britain c. 1870–1950," *History of Science*, 36 (1998), 421–68.

6   A summary volume is Charles Webster, *The National Health Service: A Political History* (Oxford: Oxford University Press, 1998).

7   Guenter Risse, *Mending Bodies, Saving Souls: A History of Hospitals* (New York: Oxford University Press, 1999).

8   *The Laboratory Revolution in Medicine*, eds Andrew Cunningham and Perry Williams (Cambridge: Cambridge University Press, 1992).

9   John Pickstone, "Medicine, Society, and the State," in *The Cambridge Illustrated History of Medicine*, ed. Roy Porter (Cambridge: Cambridge University Press, 1996), p. 304.

10 John Duffy, *From Humors to Medical Science: A History of American Medicine* (2nd edn, Urbana IL: University of Illinois Press, 1993), p. 146.

Conclusion: Where Medical History is Going

1   Charles E. Rosenberg, *Explaining Epidemics and Other Studies in the History of Medicine* (Cambridge: Cambridge University Press, 1992), especially p. 5.

2   Waltraud Ernst, "Plural Medicine, Tradition and Modernity: Historical and Contemporary Perspectives: Views from Below and from Above," in *Plural Medicine, Tradition and Modernity, 1800–2000*, ed. Waltraud Ernst (London: Routledge, 2002), p. 4.

3   Michael Neve, "Conclusion," in Lawrence I. Conrad et al., *The Western Medical Tradition, 800 BC to AD 1800* (Cambridge: Cambridge University Press, 1995), p. 477.

4   Rosemary A. Stevens, "Public Roles for the Medical Profession in the United States: Beyond Theories of Decline and Fall," *Milbank Quarterly*, 79 (2001), 327–53.

5   Virginia Berridge, "Public or Policy Understanding of History," *Social History of Medicine*, 16 (2003), 518.

6   Mark Jackson, "Disease and Diversity in History," *Social History of Medicine*, 15 (2002), 325.

Index